WILLIE & ANNIE NELSON'S
CANNABIS COOKBOOK

WILLIE&ANNIE NELSON'S CANNABIS COOKBOOK

MOUTHWATERING RECIPES & THE HIGH-FLYING STORIES BEHIND THEM

WILLIE & ANNIE NELSON

WITH DAVID RITZ, MIA TANGREDI
&
CHEF ANDREA DRUMMER

GALLERY BOOKS
NEW YORK   LONDON   TORONTO   SYDNEY   NEW DELHI

Gallery Books
An Imprint of Simon & Schuster, LLC
1230 Avenue of the Americas
New York, NY 10020

First Gallery Books hardcover edition November 2024

GALLERY BOOKS and colophon are registered trademarks of Simon & Schuster, LLC

Simon & Schuster: Celebrating 100 Years of Publishing in 2024

For information about special discounts for bulk purchases, please contact Simon & Schuster Special Sales at 1-866-506-1949 or business@simonandschuster.com.

The Simon & Schuster Speakers Bureau can bring authors to your live event. For more information or to book an event, contact the Simon & Schuster Speakers Bureau at 1-866-248-3049 or visit our website at www.simonspeakers.com.

Interior design by Matt Ryan

Photographs by Andrea Drummer

Manufactured in China

10 9 8 7 6 5 4 3 2 1

Library of Congress Control Number: 2024938139

ISBN 978-1-6680-4343-1
ISBN 978-1-6680-4344-8 (ebook)

Dedicated to all the family farmers who cultivate the food, fiber, and fuel necessary to keep the world fed, clothed, and moving forward in a wholesome way—and to all those who make sure the hungry have access to the sustenance they require.

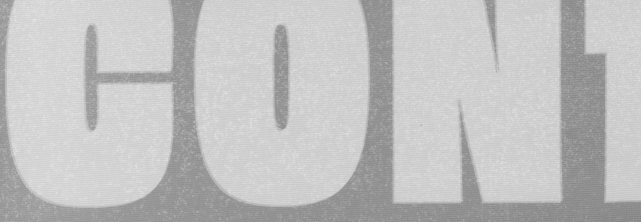

NOTE TO READER

People have different levels of familiarity and experience with ingesting cannabis. Before you begin including cannabis in your cooking, you should take note of your level of experience and make sure ingesting cannabis is right for you. Each person metabolizes THC differently. The intensity and duration of the effects can vary.

Cannabis edible consumption may cause temporary impairment of normal function. The onset of a "high" from ingesting cannabis takes longer (thirty minutes to two hours) versus the nearly instant onset from inhalation, and effects can last ten hours or more. If you have any medical conditions (physical or mental) that may be impacted by consuming cannabis-infused food, please consult your physician before ingesting. Please also note that the THC content of infused recipes requires awareness of the number of servings in a recipe and caution in portioning the meals prepared. Precautions should be taken to assure that infused foods are not consumed by children or those under the age of twenty-one. You should be aware of your local cannabis laws.

As with any THC product, it is recommended that you go slow, as the effects of THC by way of ingesting can take upwards of two hours to take effect. The ultimate outcome depends on several variables including yet not limited to your BMI and personal tolerance level and the THC content of the cannabis used for infusion.

All recipe edibles amassed in this manuscript have been created using a strain of cannabis containing 22 percent THC. Please note that using a different strain with a different percentage of THC to create oils, butters, and so on may result in an alternative result, namely a higher- or lower-dosed edible. To account for any dose adjustment, follow the recipe carefully, consider the THC percentage of the cannabis used, and label and store products according to adult use standards.

While each recipe has a specific dose, you can reduce the dosage at your discretion. It is important to note that developing a menu for a dinner by combining more than one dish containing THC will result in a high dose of THC. Please be mindful of the THC counts *per recipe* and prepare wisely. Ingesting high levels of THC can heighten your experience and create an unpleasant high. Please dose responsibly and feel free to lessen the amount of THC in any recipe.

Additional information on THC dosing is widely available.

EAT

And eating well.

Another matter altogether.

How do you define "well"?

Well, everyone would define it differently.

I'd say "well" means healthy and hearty. Eating with gusto. Eating food that hasn't been tainted with chemicals. Farm-to-table food that tastes real and right.

Cannabis is food, it's medicine, it's energy, it's health.

Without this special herb we affectionately call weed, I'd never be offering up a cookbook at age ninety-one.

Without weed and my wife, Annie, I'd probably be dead decades ago.

With weed, I'm still striving and thriving and creating new music. Not to mention having cool chefs like Andrea Drummer and Annie to cook up cannabis-flavored meals that provide nourishment, for body and soul.

Before pot, I was one of those fools who, throwing back bourbon and beer, thought I could take on the world. That meant picking on guys bigger than me. Those are the stories I'm happy to forget.

The pot stories are the ones I'm glad to remember. That's because they're good-hearted stories, mostly with happy endings.

I say "mostly" because there were, in truth, a couple of decidedly unpleasant busts. Overall, though, cannabis turned my mean to mellow. It helped me find the groove in the grind of a hectic but beautiful life of creating music.

ING...

Now I want us to help you create some beautiful food. I love the idea of incorporating cannabis into a wholesome diet. I've been a champion of its legalization since the stone ages. I couldn't be happier that the arguments advocating the many uses of the plant have finally prevailed.

Over a lifetime of study, I learned that pot is more than pleasure. Its positive properties are limitless.

It's a blessing and a blast. It's good fuel.

Together with Chef Drummer, one of the most celebrated cannabis chefs, and my wife, Annie, the most celebrated chef in our home, I'm excited to help you to cook up a whole mess of wholesome meals.

There's an abundance of information here. Abundance is the key.

An abundance of care about the food we eat.

An abundance of creativity in preparing the food.

An abundance of love in sharing the food with others.

And because I'm a storyteller by trade, an abundance of stories that carry the fragrance of the precious plant that is, after all, the centerpiece of this book.

Be patient and get to know the dosage that suits you best.

WILLIE NELSON

START LOW, GO SLOW...

I've always said that about cannabis ... well, actually I say that about life in general.

If you believe in the many benefits of cannabis, you'll want to bring folks to understand it instead of scaring them off with a bad experience, especially when it can help so many when dosed properly.

I started making edibles for my husband when he had a bad bout of pneumonia and couldn't smoke. For him it was medicine, because he needed to leave his lungs alone. I have a bit of a scientific mind and a pretty good working knowledge of the human body, so I began my mission to create an edible he would like.

Concentrating anything means you concentrate good or bad . . . always choose good. I found the best and cleanest cannabis to create my chocolates. I'm not a smoker, so creating an edible to bypass the smoke was a steep learning curve for me and very much had its ups and downs.

I hadn't smoked pot since the seventies. Back then I would take a hit, laugh my ass off, and binge munchies. My only reference at the time to current pot strains was Willie offering me a hit and me thinking it was going to be a fun afternoon. I spent it asleep because bed was the only place safe enough for me while it wore off. Yes . . . I'm a supreme lightweight!

So when I started developing edibles for him, I focused on a dose that would find a happy medium, knowing he had a sweet tooth and would likely eat more than one.

The experience was hysterical at times. One night after having finally gotten the five simple ingredients perfected, I slipped into bed, maybe a little too high. Not wanting to wake him because sleep is so good, I lay there vacillating between "OMG I'm waaaaaay too high," to laughing so hard and trying not to wake him. In the end, I'd found a great dose, and he became my guinea pig from then on. Turns out everyone loved the ones Willie taste-tested for me.

A friend was going to travel and had anxiety so asked for some chocolate to help through the flight. Willie gave him some. Turns out this "friend" had an edible company and wanted mine. We didn't agree on ingredients, but it started people coming to us with business proposals. That's the genesis of us getting into the cannabis business. We named the company Willie's Reserve. I've used my base and made other bases in many recipes and always enjoy Andrea Drummer's . . . always.

I'm celiac and have friends with glucose issues, so my edibles needed to be gluten-free with an even glycemic level. Cooking gluten-free is not difficult. Ingredients can be substituted easy enough in all recipes without compromising the integrity of a dish, including flours, sauces, and condiments. I hope you find adventure and always remember the basics.

Have fun and remember to never dose anyone . . . it's unkind, turns them off unnecessarily, and breaks our Nelson family rules of:

Don't Be an Asshole
Don't Be an Asshole
Don't Be a G-Damn Asshole.

ANNIE NELSON

A NOTE FROM CHEF ANDREA

My career as a cannabis chef began out of sheer necessity.

If you're at all familiar with the grueling work of cooks the world over, you understand the toll it can take on one's body. Oblivious to this truth, my reality check came after one year in the kitchen and in the form of sciatica.

After several prescriptions of opiates literally flushed down the toilet, I began experimenting with infusing food with cannabis as an alternative to living with chronic pain.

My intention for myself was the same as I share in these recipes: to make cannabis cuisine safe, accessible, and easy.

While consuming too much THC (tetrahydrocannabinol) will do no harm to the body, the ramifications can prove unpleasant. To that end, brands are creating safely packaged products with easy dosing directions. In addition, trained chefs are introducing recipes suitable for regular use and that integrate easily into your lifestyle.

On average the legal single dose of THC equates to 10 milligrams per serving.

This book contains recipes that make it easy to tailor the dosage to the individual using simple mathematics. The THC component can also be eliminated altogether for a family-friendly meal that's just as appetizing.

Dosages in the recipes range from 8% THC to 46% THC per serving. The intent is to present the possibilities and to acknowledge varied tolerances. The number of milligrams one should consume is contingent upon a number of factors:

- Body weight
- Metabolism

- Tolerance
- Dosage
- Type of edibles

Other factors to consider are the strains of cannabis used, the maturation process of the plant, and your overall experience with edibles. Since the body metabolizes THC differently through the liver (eating) than it does through the lungs (smoking), the experience can vary from person to person. For most, the effects last longer. For some, they are more intense.

To simplify edible THC consumption, the standard recommendation is as follows:

- **1 to 2.5 milligrams** is considered a **MICRODOSE**.
- **3 to 5 milligrams** is **LOW DOSAGE.**
- **10 TO 15 MILLIGRAMS** is **MODERATE.**
- **20 TO 30 MILLIGRAMS** is **HIGH.**
- **50 TO 100 MILLIGRAMS** is **ACUTE**.
- **100 to 500 milligrams** is considered **MACRODOSING**.

My recommendation would be the same as I adhered to when first using edibles for medicinal application: *Start low and exert patience*. And you can easily adjust the dosage in the recipes in the book.

And most important, enjoy!

CALCULATING THC DOSAGE

1 gram of cannabis = **1,000 milligrams**

10% of **1,000 milligrams** is **100 milligrams**

This means that one gram of cannabis contains 100 milligrams of THC.

Next, calculate how many milligrams are in a batch of marijuana butter. As an example, it takes one ounce (equaling 28 grams) of average quality marijuana to make one cup of butter. That would mean 2,800 milligrams of THC went into that one cup of butter.

Moving on, the amount of THC in a given recipe will depend on the amount of butter used.

If ½ cup of that butter is used to make a batch of thirty-six cookies, then the entire batch would contain 1,400 milligrams. Divide 1,400 mg by the number of servings, in this case 36, to determine that each cookie will contain about 38.8 milligrams of THC.

To recap, estimate the percentage of THC in your plant material first (or use the numbers from the lab test) and divide that into 1,000 to get the per milligram amount. Next, calculate the number of milligrams in your infusion and in the amount of infusion you will use to make your recipe. Divide that by the number of servings your recipe makes, and you will know the per serving dose.

Notably, there are convenient tools that you might use to calculate THC for dosing edibles such as the Marijuana Dosing Calculator, the Edible Dose Calculator, or the THC Calculator.

It's also important to keep in mind that THC degrades at temperatures exceeding 392°F.

BUTTER

All the following recipes for cannabis oils and butters were developed using MAC cannabis strain, which contains 22% THC. Oils and butters are interchangeable in every recipe. Keep in mind, however, that switching them may alter the flavor profile or texture. MAC, also known as Miracle Alien Cookies, is a hybrid strain that produces creative, happy, and uplifting effects. Medicinally, it is associated with alleviating stress, anxiety, and depression. MAC presents notes of orange, as well as other citrus profiles, and finishes with pepper undertones.

S&OILS

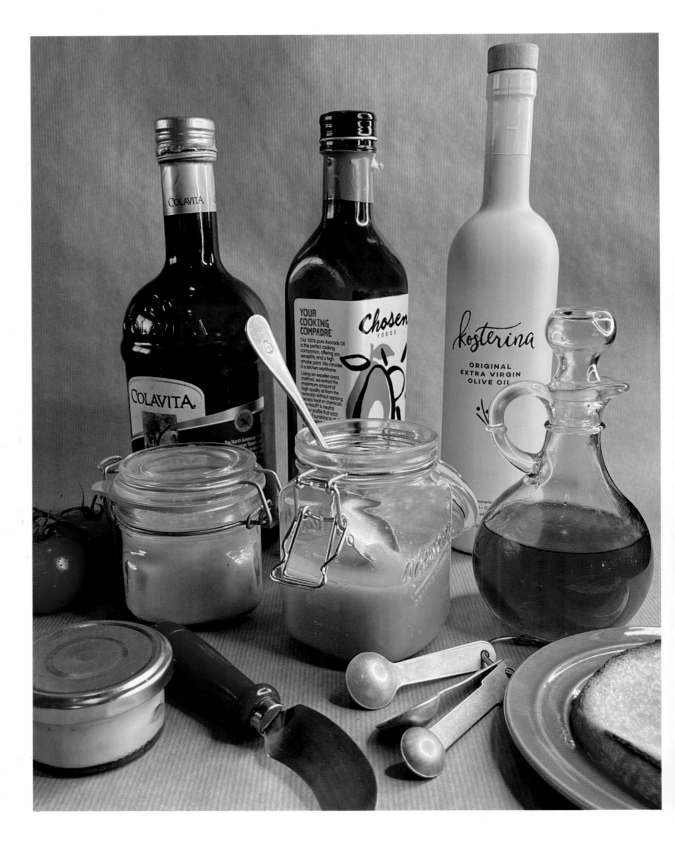

CANNABIS GHEE

MAKES **2 CUPS CANNABIS GHEE** (32 TABLESPOONS)
YIELDS **212 MG PER TABLESPOON**

28.3 grams (1 ounce) cannabis product
1 pound unsalted ghee
Cheesecloth
Kitchen twine

1 Use a coffee grinder or blender to process the cannabis product to a medium to fine grind.

2 Place the ground cannabis in layered cheesecloth and fold or bundle into a sachet. Secure tightly with kitchen twine.

3 In a 2-quart-saucepan, melt the ghee over low heat. Add the sachet and cook for 3 hours over low heat to extract the THC. Stir occasionally. DO NOT allow the ghee to reach boiling temperature.

4 Gently squeeze through a cheesecloth and cool fully before refrigerating.

VEGAN CANNABIS BUTTER

MAKES **2 CUPS CANNABIS BUTTER** (32 TABLESPOONS)
YIELDS **212 MG THC PER TABLESPOON**

28.3 grams (1 ounce) cannabis product
1 pound vegan butter
Cheesecloth
Kitchen twine

1 Use a coffee grinder or blender to process the cannabis product into a fine to medium grind.

2 Place the ground cannabis in layered cheesecloth and fold or bundle into a sachet. Secure tightly with kitchen twine.

3 In a 2-quart saucepan, melt the butter over low heat. Add the sachet and cook for 1½ hours over low heat to extract the THC. Stir occasionally. DO NOT allow the butter to reach boiling temperature.

4 Gently squeeze through cheesecloth. Cool fully before refrigerating.

CANNABIS AVOCADO OIL

MAKES **4 CUPS CANNABIS OIL** (64 TABLESPOONS)
YIELDS **141 MG THC PER TABLESPOON**

28.3 grams (1 ounce)
   cannabis product

Cheesecloth

Kitchen twine

32 fluid ounces (1 quart)
   high-temperature
   avocado oil

1 Use a coffee grinder or blender to process the cannabis product to a medium to fine grind.

2 Place the ground cannabis in layered cheesecloth and fold or bundle into a sachet. Secure tightly with kitchen twine.

3 In a 2-quart saucepan, combine the oil and cannabis sachet and cook for 1½ to 2 hours over low heat to extract the THC. Stir occasionally. DO NOT allow the oil to reach boiling temperature.

4 Cool, and squeeze through a cheesecloth. Store in a cool dry place or in the refrigerator.

CANNABIS COCONUT OIL

MAKES **4 CUPS CANNABIS OIL** (64 TABLESPOONS)
YIELDS **141 MG THC PER TABLESPOON**

28.3 grams (1 ounce)
   cannabis product

Cheesecloth

Kitchen twine

32 fluid ounces (1 quart)
   high-temperature
   coconut oil

1 Use a coffee grinder or blender to process the cannabis product to a medium to fine grind.

2 Place the ground cannabis in layered cheesecloth and fold or bundle into a sachet. Secure tightly with kitchen twine.

NOTE: The cannabis-infused coconut oil can also be used as a topical.

3 In a 2-quart saucepan, combine the oil and cannabis sachet and cook for 1½ to 2 hours over low heat to extract the THC. Stir occasionally. DO NOT allow the oil to reach boiling temperature.

4 Cool, and gently squeeze through cheesecloth. Store in a cool, dry place or in the refrigerator.

CANNABIS GRAPESEED OIL

MAKES **4 CUPS CANNABIS OIL** (64 TABLESPOONS)
YIELDS **141 MG THC PER TABLESPOON**

28.3 grams (1 ounce) cannabis product
Cheesecloth
Kitchen twine
32 fluid ounces (1 quart) high-temperature grapeseed oil

1 Use a coffee grinder or blender to process the cannabis product to a medium to fine grind.

2 Place the ground cannabis in layered cheesecloth and fold or bundle into a sachet. Secure tightly with kitchen twine.

3 In a 2-quart saucepan, combine the oil and cannabis sachet and cook for 1½ to 2 hours over low heat to extract the THC. Stir occasionally. DO NOT allow the oil to reach boiling temperature.

4 Cool. Gently squeeze though cheesecloth and discard cannabis. Store in a cool dry place or in the refrigerator.

BAR C
&
HONKY

RAWLS

&

TONKS

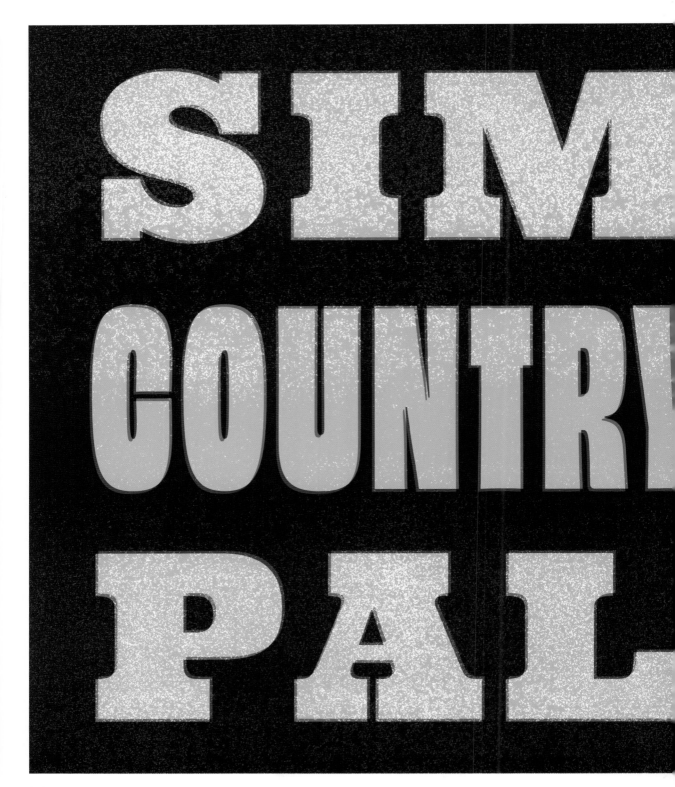

PLE BOY PLATE

When it comes to food, I like the basics: beans and cornbread, tacos, bacon and eggs, bacon and waffles, and sausage and eggs. The simple things always bring me the most happiness, but I step out of the box now and again and enjoy new and different meals. In this book you'll find both. I hope you try the simple recipes we often enjoy at home, as well as the more complex variations created by our favorite cannabis chef, Andrea Drummer.

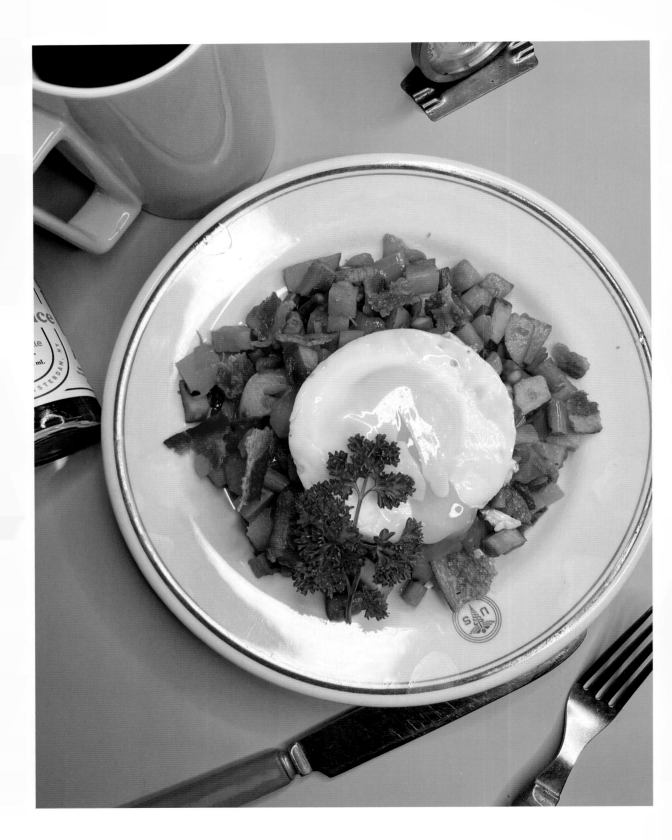

WILLIE'S FAVORITE SWEET POTATO HASH WITH FARM FRESH EGGS & APPLEWOOD-SMOKED BACON

MAKES **4 SERVINGS**
17.6 MG THC PER SERVING

¼ pound applewood-smoked bacon, diced

1 medium yellow onion, cut into medium dice

1 large russet potato, cut into medium dice

1 large sweet potato, cut into medium dice

½ pound asparagus, cut into ¼-inch pieces

½ red bell pepper, diced

Olive oil

½ teaspoon Cannabis Grapeseed Oil (page 11)

Coarse sea salt

8 farm-fresh eggs

1 In a large cast-iron skillet, cook the diced bacon over medium heat until crispy. Transfer the bacon to a plate, leaving the rendered fat behind in the skillet.

2 Add the onion to the bacon fat in the skillet and cook until translucent.

3 Add the russet potato and sweet potato and stir until the ingredients are integrated. Continue to cook and stir occasionally until the potatoes are al dente.

4 Add the asparagus and bell pepper. Add olive oil to the pan if necessary. Cook until the vegetables are tender and the potatoes are completely cooked through.

continues

WILLIE'S FAVORITE SWEET POTATO HASH WITH FARM FRESH EGGS & APPLEWOOD-SMOKED BACON
continued

5 Remove from the heat. Return the crispy bacon to the skillet and add the cannabis grapeseed oil. Mix until evenly incorporated. Season to taste with coarse sea salt. Set aside.

6 In a separate cast-iron skillet, warm a generous amount of olive oil over medium-low heat. Crack 4 eggs into the skillet, cover, and cook until the egg whites are solid and the yolk is still runny. Repeat with the remaining 4 eggs and more olive oil.

7 To plate, portion out the hash evenly onto four plates. Top each with 2 eggs and finish with a pinch of coarse sea salt.

POTATO RÖSTI

MAKES **2 SERVINGS**
5.2 MG PER SERVING

3 Yukon Gold potatoes, peeled and coarsely grated

1 shallot, finely diced

1 medium egg, beaten, or equivalent egg replacer

¼ teaspoon Cannabis Avocado Oil (page 10)

1 teaspoon finely chopped fresh sage

1 teaspoon granulated garlic

1 teaspoon all-purpose flour

1 teaspoon mustard powder

¼ teaspoon baking powder

Kosher salt and freshly ground black pepper

3 tablespoons neutral oil

FOR SERVING
Sour cream
Chopped fresh chives
Flaky sea salt

1 Squeeze any excess water out of the grated potatoes. Transfer to a bowl and add the shallot, egg, cannabis oil, chopped sage, granulated garlic, flour, mustard powder, baking powder, and salt and pepper to taste. Mix until well combined.

2 In a medium skillet, heat the neutral oil over medium heat. Divide the rösti mixture into 4 equal portions. Spoon the mixture into the hot pan and flatten with the back of the spoon. Cook until golden brown and crisp, about 5 minutes per side. Drain on paper towels.

3 To serve: plate 2 rösti per person and accompany with sour cream, chopped chives, and flaky salt.

CHEF'S NOTES: This pairs perfectly with Vegan Carrot Lox (page 20) and Zeroe brand plant-based caviar.

VEGAN CARROT LOX

MAKES **10 SERVINGS**
14.1 MG PER SERVING

4 large carrots, peeled

¾ cup hot water

¼ cup liquid smoke

3 tablespoons caper brine

3 tablespoons soy sauce or tamari

2 tablespoons rice vinegar

1 tablespoon vegan fish sauce

1 tablespoon white miso

1 tablespoon kelp granules

1 tablespoon garlic powder

1 teaspoon fine sea salt

1 teaspoon fresh lemon juice

¼ cup good-quality olive oil, preferably Kosterina Greek olive oil

½ tablespoon Cannabis Grapeseed Oil (page 11)

1 teaspoon Maldon flaky sea salt, for garnish

CHEF'S NOTE: Serve with toasted bagels, Potato Rösti (page 19), or with tomato cucumber salad.

1 Use a vegetable peeler to create carrot ribbons and set aside.

2 In a medium saucepan, whisk together the water, liquid smoke, caper brine, soy sauce, vinegar, fish sauce, miso, kelp granules, garlic powder, and fine sea salt. Bring to a bold simmer, over medium heat.

3 Add the carrot ribbons, cover, reduce the heat, and simmer until the carrot ribbons are supple but al dente. Be sure to monitor the cooking process to avoid your carrot lox getting mushy.

4 Remove from the heat and allow the lox to cook at room temperature. The residual heat should create the ideal consistency.

5 Once cooled, add the lemon juice and transfer to a sealed container. Marinate in the fridge overnight.

6 Remove the lox from the refrigerator and drain. Pat the lox until they are completely free of moisture. Toss with the olive oil and cannabis oil for the similar mouthfeel of fatty smoked salmon. Garnish with flaky salt.

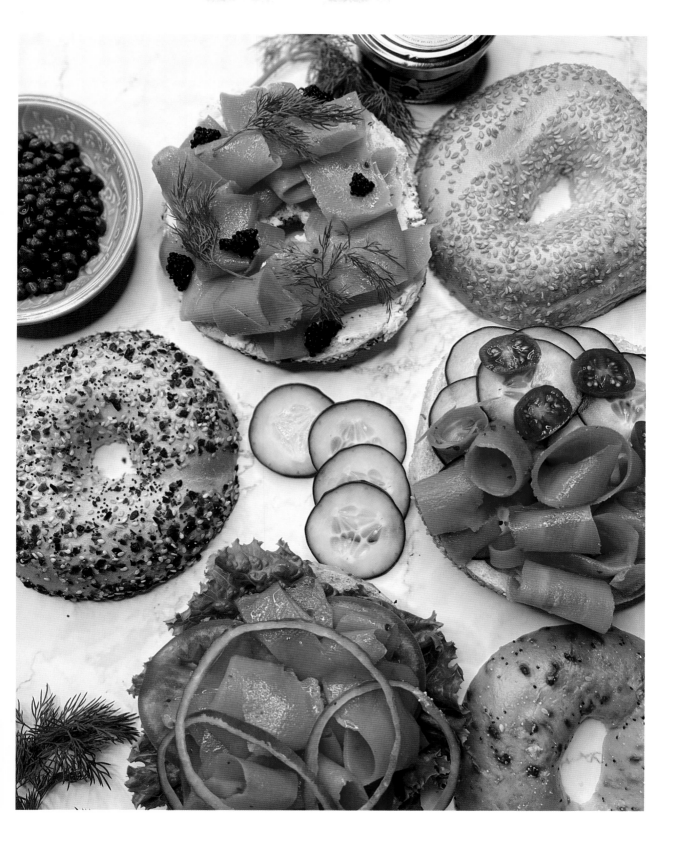

MUNCHIES

HUGE CATEGORY.

Huge delight or huge problem.

The problem can be solved by not going overboard. But not everyone can control their appetite.

I'm lucky not to be an overeater. Maybe that's why I'm delighting in this cookbook.

I also delight in the munchies. It's fun to all of a sudden get an urgent message from your belly saying, "Feed me something good, and feed me now!"

Along those lines, here are some suggestions for tasty little items that, when eaten in moderation, might make the munchies a delight for you as well.

THREE-LAYER SKILLET BROWNIES

MAKES **5 SERVINGS**
14.1 MG PER SERVING

8 tablespoons (4 ounces) butter

1 teaspoon Cannabis Ghee (page 9)

4 ounces plus ½ cup semisweet chocolate chips

1½ ounces Ghirardelli's unsweetened chocolate, chopped

2 large eggs

1½ teaspoons vanilla extract

½ cup sugar

¼ cup plus 1 tablespoon all-purpose flour

1 teaspoon baking powder

¼ teaspoon salt

½ cup toffee bits

2½ cups store bought, room temperature cookie dough

2½ cups coarsely crushed Biscoff cookies

CHEF'S NOTE: Serve warm with vanilla ice cream and warm salted caramel sauce.

1 Preheat the oven to 350°F.

2 In a large bowl set over a pan of simmering water, melt the butter, cannabis ghee, 4 ounces of the chocolate chips, and the unsweetened Ghirardelli's chocolate until smooth. Set aside and allow it to cool.

3 Meanwhile, in a large bowl, stir together the eggs, vanilla, and sugar.

4 Stir the cooled chocolate mixture into the egg mixture. Mix until well combined.

5 In a medium bowl, sift together ¼ cup of the flour, the baking powder, and salt. Add this to the chocolate mixture, stirring until combined. In a medium bowl, toss together the remaining ½ cup chocolate chips, the toffee bits, and remaining 1 tablespoon flour and fold them into the chocolate mixture.

6 Press ½ cup of cookie dough into each of five 3½-inch cast-iron skillets. Use more, if desired, to achieve an even layer.

7 Make a layer in each skillet of ½ cup Biscoff cookies. Divide the brownie batter equally among the five skillets and place on a baking sheet.

8 Cook until browned, about 25 minutes, being mindful not to overcook. Serve warm.

VEGAN BUTTER PECAN ICE CREAM

MAKES **6 CUPS**
20.1 MG PER 1 CUP SERVING

½ cup packed chopped dates

¼ cup coconut sugar

½ cup unsweetened almond milk

Pinch of sea salt

1 tablespoon Vegan Cannabis Butter (page 9)

2 tablespoons vegan butter

2¾ cups full-fat coconut milk

1 vanilla bean, split lengthwise

¾ cup pecans, coarsely chopped

1 In a small saucepan, combine the dates, coconut sugar, and almond milk and bring to a boil over medium-low heat. Remove from the heat and whisk in the sea salt, cannabis butter, and ½ tablespoon of the vegan butter.

2 Transfer the mixture to a blender, being mindful of the hot contents. Pulse first and then blend on high speed until smooth. Add the coconut milk to the blender and scrape the vanilla seeds into the date mixture. Blend until smooth.

3 Pour into a sealable jar or container and refrigerate for 8 hours or overnight.

4 Meanwhile, in a skillet, combine the chopped pecans and the remaining 1½ tablespoons vegan butter and toast over medium heat until they are golden brown. Transfer to a baking sheet to cool.

5 Give the chilled custard a shake or stir if the mixture has separated (this is normal). Pour into an ice cream maker and churn according to the manufacturer's directions. Add the toasted buttered pecans during the last 5 minutes of churning.

6 Once the ice cream has thickened and the churning process is complete, serve immediately for soft serve, or transfer it to a freezer-safe 1½- to 2-quart glass storage container and freeze for 6 hours for a firmer texture.

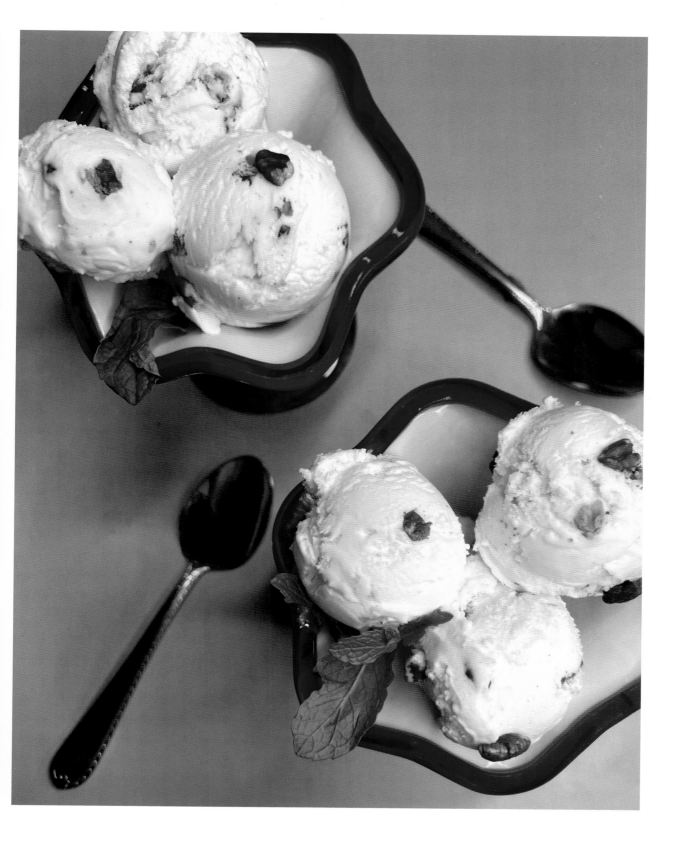

"JUST WH[EN]
YOU THI[NK]
YOU'VE B[EEN]
PATI[ENT]
ENOUGH[,]

. . . you've gotta be more patient."

I was talking to my best friend and drummer, Paul English. We were in a restaurant in Fayetteville, Arkansas, waiting for our food. It was a Sunday, the churches had just let out, and the place was jam-packed.

The aroma of good food cooking in the kitchen was making Paul a little crazy. I usually keep my philosophy to myself, but being in Arkansas, the original home of my people, put me in a reflective frame of mind. I was thinking of the fortitude it took for them to leave their home in the hills and trek down to Texas. Fortitude and patience.

Patience is a beautiful thing to cultivate. I've tried. And on that early afternoon in Fayetteville, as the smell of simmering roast and ribs had Paul on the verge of attacking the cook cause our food still hadn't arrived, I said, "Sometimes the anticipation is the sweetest part of all."

"Maybe so, Willie," said Paul, "but I still want my food. *Right now!*"

Here's a recipe that, while mouth-wateringly delicious, requires some patience. As it's cooking, here's hoping you can savor the anticipation.

BEEF SHANKS & RED-EYE GRAVY

MAKES **8 SERVINGS**
15.1 MG PER SERVING

3 tablespoons browning sauce

8 beef shanks (14 ounces each), cut 2 inches thick

2 cups all-purpose flour

Kosher salt and freshly ground black pepper

¼ cup vegetable oil, plus more if needed

1 large onion, diced

2 celery stalks, diced

2 carrots, diced

8 large garlic cloves, minced

2 large sprigs fresh thyme

1 sprig fresh rosemary

1 bay leaf

2 tablespoons tomato paste

3 cups strong black coffee

6 cups beef broth

1 tablespoon Cannabis Ghee (page 9)

1 Preheat the oven to 300°F.

2 In a bowl, with impeccably clean or gloved hands, work the browning sauce into the shanks, evenly coating each.

3 In a large bowl, season the flour with salt and pepper. Coat the beef shanks in the flour mixture, shaking off any excess flour.

4 In a large Dutch oven, heat the oil over medium heat until shimmering. Working in batches (taking care not to overcrowd the pot), brown the beef shanks on each side. Once golden, transfer the shanks to a large roasting pan and arrange in a single layer. Set aside.

5 Reduce the heat under the Dutch oven to medium to low heat. Add the onion, celery, and carrots. Add additional oil, if necessary. Stir until the onion is translucent.

6 Add the garlic, thyme, rosemary, bay leaf, and tomato paste and cook for 1 to 2 minutes, stirring continuously. Deglaze the pot with the coffee and stir to incorporate any bits at the bottom of the pot. Add the beef broth and stir until thoroughly incorporated.

7 Pour the contents of the Dutch oven over the beef shanks and cover with foil or a fitted lid. Transfer to the oven and braise until fork-tender, about 2½ hours.

8 Uncover and braise for 30 minutes longer. Transfer the shanks to a large sheet pan and cover with foil.

9 Remove the herbs stems and bay leaf and transfer the braising liquid (including vegetables) to a blender and blend until smooth.

10 Transfer the mixture to a clean pot and cook over medium-low heat until the sauce lightly coats the back of a spoon. Stir the cannabis ghee into the sauce and thoroughly incorporate.

11 Spoon the sauce over the shanks and serve hot.

"CHILI RICE IS OH SO VERY NICE"

In our Hawaii home, chili rice is a staple. When we'd go see our sons Lukas and Micah's sports games or school events, chili rice was always in the mix.

This dish also reminds me of Shanghai Jimmy, a character whose travels to the Far East were documented in newspaper clippings and journal entries on the walls of his downtown Dallas eatery on Live Oak Street. It was a tiny joint where the best item—Double Number 9—consisted of a quart-size tub of steaming rice covered with chili, cheese, raw onions, and a huge chunk of butter. If memory serves me right, it cost a buck.

These were the late fifties when Dallas was smack in the middle of its uptight *Mad Men* phase. Ninety-five percent of Jimmy's customers were guys on their lunch break from the ad agencies, banks, and insurance firms that dominated the area. They wore the uniform of the day: dark suit, white shirt, conventional tie.

Jimmy's uniform was anything but conventional. He liked parading around in his dirty jeans and chili-smeared apron. I think Jimmy liked me because I was different. I liked him for the same reason. He told me about the times that Elvis came in to grab a Double Number 9. Did I believe him? Sure. Everyone loved Jimmy's chili rice. Why would Elvis be any different?

In the age of maximum conformity, Shanghai Jimmy had his own system of survival: make his signature dish so damn delicious that he could keep his place as funky as he wanted. And believe me, both the man and his food were the essence of soulful good-feeling funk.

NIGERIAN SUYA SPICED CHILI

MAKES **4 SERVINGS**
11.7 MG PER SERVING

2 tablespoons neutral oil

1 pound beef stew meat, cubed

1 teaspoon Cannabis Avocado Oil (page 10)

1 onion, diced

2 red bell peppers, diced

4 garlic cloves, minced

1 teaspoon minced Scotch bonnet pepper

1 teaspoon ground cumin

1 tablespoon tomato paste

3 tablespoons suya spice blend (see Note)

Pinch kosher salt

1 (14.5-ounce) can diced tomatoes

2 bay leaves

1 cup veal or beef stock

1 cup dried oloyin honey beans (see Note), washed

2 tablespoons olive oil

FOR SERVING

Cooked rice

2 cups grilled onions

3 Roma (plum) tomatoes, seeded and diced

Chopped fresh parsley, for garnish

CHEF'S NOTE: Suya spice blend is used to season the Nigerian beef dish called suya. And ewa oloyin (honey beans) are a small Nigerian bean similar to black-eyed peas. Both are easily found online, and anywhere African ingredients are sold.

1 In a large Dutch oven, heat the neutral oil over medium heat until shimmering. Add the stew beef chunks and cook until browned on all sides. Transfer to a bowl and set aside.

2 Add the cannabis oil to the pan and allow it to heat up. Add the onion, bell peppers, garlic, Scotch bonnet, cumin, and tomato paste. Stir to evenly coat the vegetables with the tomato paste.

3 Return the meat to the pot along with the suya spice and kosher salt. Stir and cook for 1 to 3 minutes, until the spice is toasted and fragrant. Stir in the canned tomatoes and bay leaves. Add the veal stock, reduce the heat to a simmer, and cook uncovered for 1½ hours.

4 Stir in the beans, cover, and cook until the beans are tender, about 30 minutes.

5 Serve over rice with grilled onions, diced tomatoes, and chopped parsley.

HERE'S TO ALL THE WAITRESSES & WAITERS

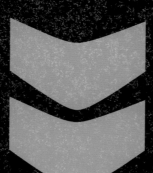

My first wife, Martha Jewel Mathews, a full-blooded Cherokee, and my current wife, Annie, a full-blooded Italian, were both waitresses; both sassy and pretty and forces of endless energy. Like all successful food servers, they had the right set of skills: Don't be afraid to smile, be friendly, look your customer in the eye, and be patient. If they need time to order, wait, be sharp, and be aware if a customer is in a hurry and needs the check.

So a big tip of my hat to all those brave souls who break their backs bringing us food, whether in some fancy bistro or a dive back of town. It's noble work.

World traveler/food connoisseur/chef Anthony Bourdain put it best:

"IF YOU'RE A CHEAP TIPPER OR RUDE TO YOUR SERVER, YOU ARE DEAD TO ME. YOU ARE LOWER THAN WHALE FECES."

"BLOODY MARY MORNIN

This is one my better-known songs. Another song I sing almost every show is "Whiskey River." I didn't write it—my friend Johnny Bush did—but I love singing it. Both are about using booze to numb heartache and pain.

An old friend, who knew me from my days in Waco, asked me about it. "Willie," he said, "you're always talking about how booze nearly ruined you and how pot saved you." He said, "So, don't you feel hypocritical about singing all these whiskey songs?"

Straight up: "No." Everyone has their thing and I am no one to judge. I'm not a preacher and I'm not a proselytizer. I don't tell folks how to live their lives. Whiskey works for some people, and others abuse it. Same with weed. My personal journey is my story. But it isn't everyone's.

Every song I sing isn't the story of my life. I invent characters who aren't me and I sing other people's songs and their truths; songs written by everyone from George Gershwin to Dolly Parton. I believe that's what a true artist tries to do—travel beyond themselves. I might not drink a Bloody Mary, but I know a good recipe when I taste one. Careful, this one has some spice.

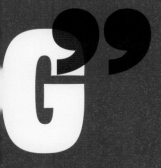

EMBOLDENED BLOODY MARY

MAKES **48 OUNCES**
30 MG PER 4-OUNCE SERVING

BLOODY MARY MIX

- 6 cups canned whole San Marzano tomatoes
- ¾ cup Clamato juice
- 3 tablespoons Worcestershire sauce
- 1 tablespoon garlic salt
- 2¼ teaspoons celery salt
- ½ teaspoon Tabasco sauce
- 1 tablespoon freshly ground black pepper
- 1.5 grams ground Watermelon Zkittlez cannabis, (24%) tied in a cheesecloth sachet
- 3 tablespoons creamy horseradish

ASSEMBLY

- 1 tablespoon celery salt
- 1 tablespoon kosher salt
- Lemon wedges
- Ice
- Tonic water
- Vodka (optional)
- Celery sticks, for garnish
- Stuffed olives, for garnish

1 MAKE THE BLOODY MARY MIX: In a large saucepan, combine the tomatoes, 2 cups water, the Clamato juice, Worcestershire sauce, garlic salt, celery salt, Tabasco sauce, black pepper, and cannabis sachet. Cook over medium-high heat for 10 minutes. Reduce the temperature and simmer over low heat for an additional 20 minutes; if too thick, add more water to achieve desired consistency.

2 Remove from the heat and allow the mixture to cool. Strain and discard the cannabis sachet.

3 Using an immersion blender or handheld mixer, blend the ingredients until smooth. Add the creamy horseradish and mix until well incorporated.

4 TO ASSEMBLE DRINKS: On a small plate, mix the celery salt and kosher salt. Moisten the rim of a glass with a lemon wedge, then dip into the salt mix and twist.

5 Fill an 8-ounce glass to the top with ice. Add 2 ounces tonic water and 1 ounce vodka if desired. Top with 4 ounces of Bloody Mary mix.

6 Garnish with celery sticks, a lemon wedge, and a speared stuffed olive.

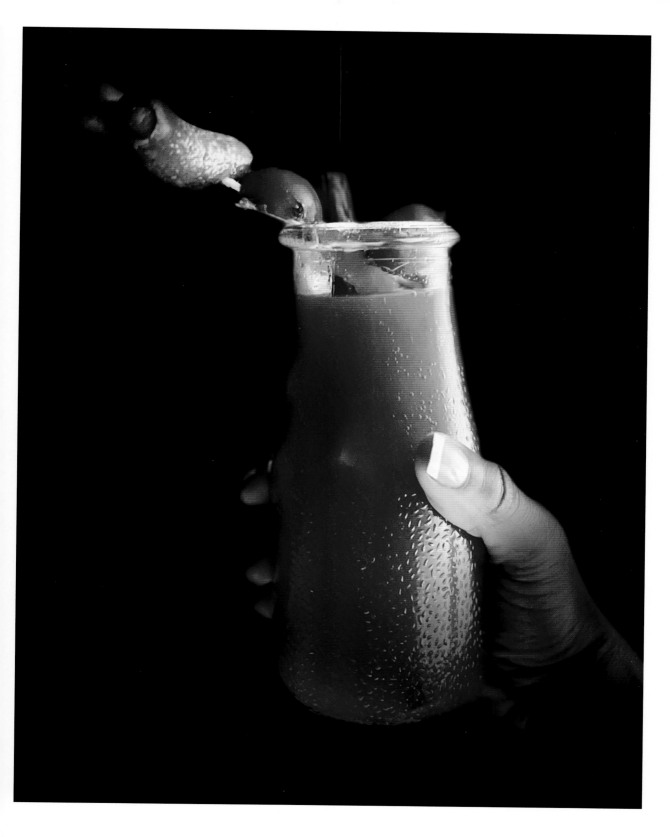

WAYLON & THE HIPPIES IN HARMONY

The Age of Aquarius was still going strong.

I was living in Austin and playing the Armadillo World Headquarters, commonly known as the Dillo.

It was hippie headquarters where artists like New Riders of the Purple Sage, Commander Cody and His Lost Pilot Airmen, and the Lost Gonzo Band found their way to favor.

The Dillo welcomed me with open arms and became one of my main go-to venues.

Waylon Jennings, a Texan himself, came to see what the fuss was all about. He viewed hippies as an alien culture.

"Then I'm an alien myself," I said.

Waylon laughed but remained skeptical. He was sure this new generation wouldn't go for his music. I was sure they would.

"Give it a try," I urged.

He tried and triumphed. Seven encores. Ol' Waylon was so happy he said he'd buy me dinner.

I took him up on it. We were both serious lovers of Tex-Mex cuisine.

This recipe isn't exactly the dish we ate, but believe you me, it'll do.

TEX-MEX GUACAMOLE

MAKES **10 SERVINGS**
14 MG PER SERVING

TACO SEASONING

1 teaspoon dried oregano

½ teaspoon chili powder

½ teaspoon ground cumin

½ teaspoon garlic powder

½ teaspoon sweet paprika

½ teaspoon kosher salt

GUACAMOLE

4 avocados, halved and pitted

Juice of 1 lime

3 garlic cloves, minced

1 tablespoon Cannabis Avocado Oil (page 10)

¼ cup corn kernels, pan seared

¼ cup cooked or canned black beans

¼ cup diced red onion

1 jalapeño, finely chopped

1 Roma tomato, finely chopped

¼ cup chopped fresh cilantro

1 MAKE THE TACO SEASONING: In a small bowl, mix together the oregano, chili powder, cumin, garlic powder, paprika, and salt. Set aside.

2 MAKE THE GUACAMOLE: Scoop the avocado into a large bowl and mash with a fork or potato masher until smooth or to achieve your desired texture.

3 Add the lime juice, taco seasoning, and minced garlic and mix well. Add the cannabis oil, corn, black beans, red onion, jalapeño, tomato, and cilantro and mix.

4 Adjust seasoning as desired.

CHEF'S NOTES: Serve with tortillas or on breakfast toast with egg and chili oil.

Double or triple the spices for the taco seasoning and keep the extra on hand.

SOUTHWEST VEGAN LOBSTER ROLLS

MAKES **8 SERVINGS**
17.6 MG PER SERVING

5 (14-ounce) cans hearts of palm, undrained

¼ cup soy sauce

¼ cup vegan fish sauce

3 tablespoons powdered beet or 1½ tablespoons organic red food coloring

1 tablespoon apple cider vinegar

½ cup vegan mayonnaise

½ teaspoon chipotle sauce

2 tablespoons vegan butter

1 tablespoon minced garlic

1 cup fresh corn kernels, roasted on the cob and cut from the cob

1 cup diced celery

2 tablespoons diced red onion

¾ cup pickled sliced jalapeños

2 tablespoons chopped fresh cilantro

1 tablespoon Cannabis Avocado Oil (page 10)

Kosher or sea salt

ASSEMBLY

8 vegan brioche buns or hot dog rolls, split

Vegan butter, melted

Diced avocado

Lemon wedges, for squeezing

1 Drain the brine from the hearts of palm into a saucepan. Add the soy sauce, vegan fish sauce, beet powder, and vinegar and whisk until fully combined. Cook over medium heat for 1 minute, then remove from the heat.

2 Transfer the hearts of palm to a glass dish and pour the marinade over them until they are fully submerged. Let cool to room temperature, cover, and refrigerate overnight.

3 In a small bowl, mix the mayonnaise and chipotle sauce together. Refrigerate the chipotle mayonnaise until ready to serve.

4 In a small saucepan, heat the vegan butter over medium heat. Add the garlic and stir for about 1 minute or until fragrant. Set aside to cool.

5 Remove the hearts of palm from the refrigerator and drain. Pat dry and chop them into bite-size pieces, replicating chopped lobster.

continues

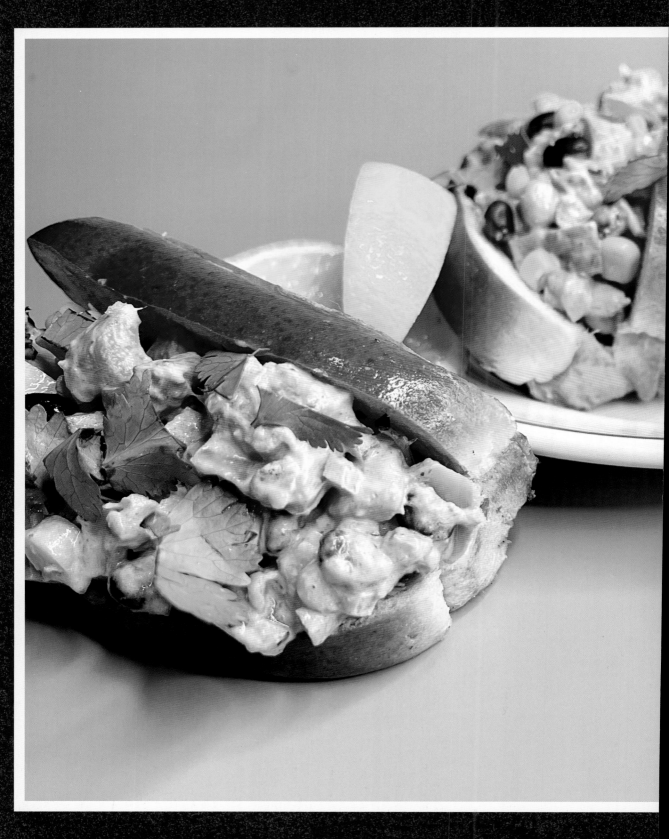

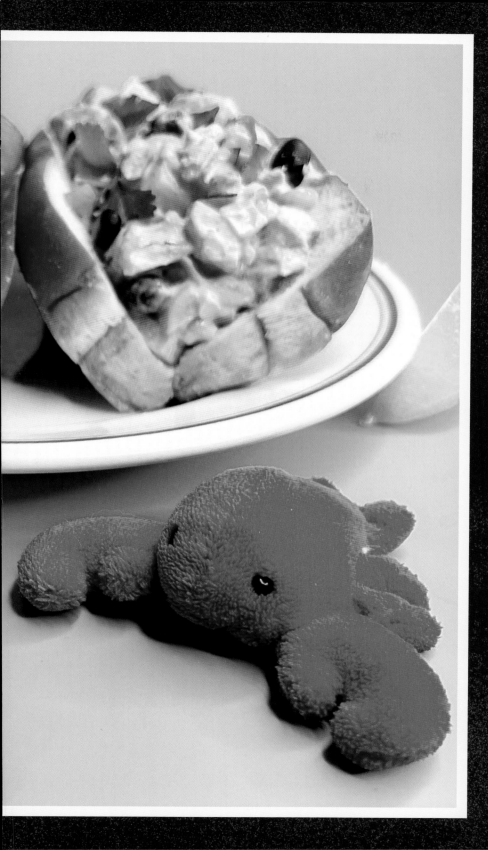

SOUTHWEST VEGAN LOBSTER ROLL
continued

6 In a bowl, toss together the sautéed garlic, roasted corn, celery, red onion, pickled jalapeño, cilantro, cannabis oil, and chipotle mayonnaise. Fold together until well combined. Season with kosher salt to taste and refrigerate until ready to assemble.

7 TO ASSEMBLE: Brush the brioche buns with the melted vegan butter and toast in the oven until golden.

8 Add equal amounts of the "lobster" mixture to each toasted roll. Finish with diced avocado and serve with lemon wedges.

CONFES OF A CARN

I love animals, but I never converted to vegetarianism. Probably would have, but the way I was raised formed my culinary habits early on. And my taste for a pork chop and good steak never went away.

Texas is cattle country. Prime cuts came much later in life, but the basic burger was part of my rural upbringing. The basic burger remains a staple of American life.

Me and Paul were once talking to a character I'll call Killer Kelly, a notorious Ft. Worth denizen who'd spent years in the Big House. He'd seen many of those "dead man walking" ordeals when prisoners were escorted to the chair that no one ever wants to sit in.

"When it was time for their last meal," he said, "the order was always the same."

SSIONS

IVORE

"A juicy cheeseburger and a mountain of fries," Paul guessed.

"You guessed right," Killer acknowledged.

Killer was telling us all this as we sat at the counter of a joint close to the stockyards. The joint was famous for its smoky ambience and flavorful burgers. That brought Killer's story closer to home.

I took a bite of my burger and thought that, hell, as a last meal, this wouldn't be a bad bet.

The noble combination of burger and fries has been refined and re-refined more times than anyone can count.

Here's one approach that, for my money, is so tasty you may well wind up agreeing with those poor souls memorialized by Killer Kelly.

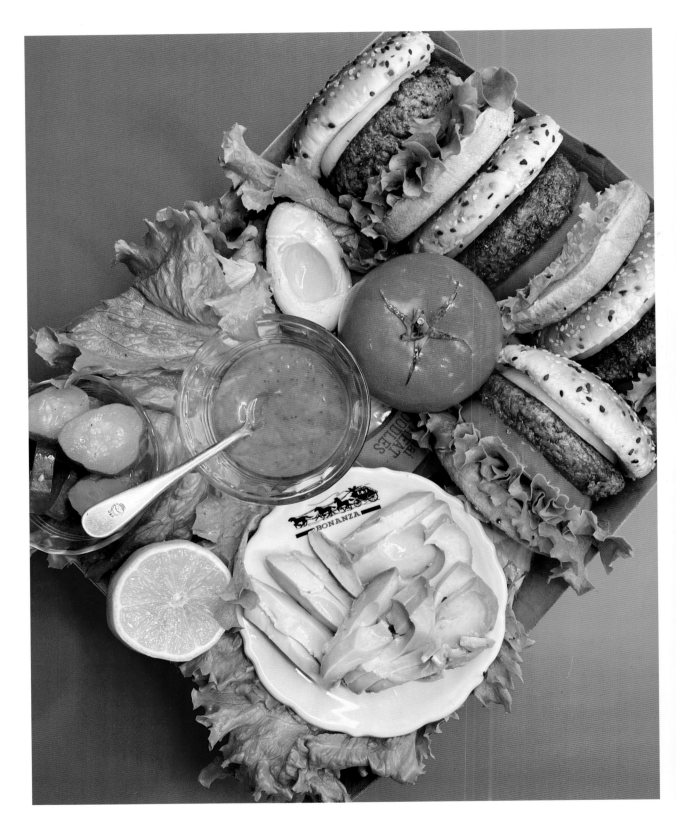

THE 50/50 BURGER

MAKES **8 BURGERS**

7.9 MG PER BURGER WITH CURRY KETCHUP

1 pound ground beef

1 pound trimmed duck thigh meat, ground (see Note)

2 tablespoons olive oil

2 tablespoons Worcestershire sauce

1 teaspoon garlic powder

1½ teaspoons kosher salt

1 teaspoon freshly ground black pepper

CHEF'S NOTE: For a richer burger, grind a few ounces of the trimmed duck fat along with the meat of the thighs.

ASSEMBLY

8 slices aged cheddar cheese

8 Röckenwagner Pretzel Buns, split

Scant ½ cup Curry Ketchup (recipe follows)

Bread and butter pickles

Optional toppings: tomato, lettuce, onion, bacon

1 In a large bowl, combine the beef, duck, olive oil, Worcestershire sauce, garlic powder, salt, and pepper. With impeccably clean hands, mix the ingredients together, taking care not to overwork the meat.

2 Divide into 8 equal portions (about 4 ounces each) and shape into ½-inch-thick patties. Using your thumb, make a single indentation in the center of each patty to prevent bulging.

3 Preheat a large cast-iron skillet over medium-high heat. Add 4 burgers, cover, and cook until browned on the bottom, 4 to 5 minutes. Do not move or press burgers.

4 Flip and top with a slice of cheese and cook to desired doneness (see doneness and timing chart below). Remove the burgers and allow them to rest for a few minutes before serving.

5 Repeat the process until all 8 patties are cooked to perfection.

6 Slide a burger into a pretzel bun and top each with a scant tablespoon of the curry ketchup. Serve with pickles and any additional toppings.

DONENESS	TEMPERATURE (°F)	COOKING TIME
RARE	120° TO 125°F	4 TO 5 MINUTES
MEDIUM-RARE	130° TO 135°F	5 TO 6 MINUTES
MEDIUM	140° TO 145°F	6 TO 8 MINUTES
MEDIUM-WELL	150° TO 155°F	8 TO 9 MINUTES
WELL-DONE	160° TO 165°F	9 TO 10 MINUTES

CURRY KETCHUP

MAKES **1 CUP** (16 TABLESPOONS)
7.9 MG PER SCANT 1 TABLESPOON

1 tablespoon Cannabis Avocado Oil (page 10) or Cannabis Grapeseed Oil (page 11)

1 medium onion, diced

2 garlic cloves, minced

7 ounces tomato paste (about ¾ cup)

2 tablespoons agave syrup

1 tablespoon distilled white vinegar

1 teaspoon curry powder

1 teaspoon kosher salt, or to taste

1 In a skillet, heat the cannabis oil over medium heat. Add the onion and garlic and cook until the onion is translucent.

2 Add the tomato paste and sauté briefly, then add ⅔ cup water to deglaze the pan. Bring the mixture to a boil. Add the agave, vinegar, curry powder, and salt and boil 5 to 7 minutes.

3 Transfer the mixture to a small blender and process until you achieve the desired smoothness. Adjust the seasoning and store in a sealable container in the refrigerator.

GOTTA LOVE BAR FOOD

All food has its place. Each category of food contains good and bad dishes, and naturally I'm interested in promoting the good. A lot of bar food isn't too good. That's because such establishments put booze first and food second. As Mark Twain said, "All generalizations are false, including this one." That brings me to an exception to the generalization.

I hope my memory is clear because, to be honest, this was something I discovered on tour somewhere in the great state of Wisconsin. I found a bar where the food was so tasty that I forgot about the booze. Of course, Wisconsin is famous for cheese, and the grilled cheese sandwich was memorable. Was it swiss? Was it cheddar? Was it parmesan? Maybe all three . . . with the bread toasted to a buttery brown. I still hold that image of the cheese oozing over the crust.

HERB-CRUSTED GRILLED CHEESE

MAKES **4 SANDWICHES**
10.4 MG PER SANDWICH

6 tablespoons
mayonnaise

4 tablespoons Dijon
mustard

1 ounce minced fresh
thyme

1 ounce minced fresh
rosemary

1 ounce minced fresh
oregano

1 ounce minced fresh
basil

8 slices artisan,
French, or
sourdough bread

4 ounces Camembert
cheese

1 teaspoon Cannabis
Ghee (page 9), at
room temperature
(see Note)

2 teaspoons freshly
ground black
pepper

12 ounces Gruyère
cheese, grated, at
room temperature

6 ounces white
cheddar cheese,
grated, at room
temperature

16 slices firm-ripe
heirloom tomatoes

CHEF'S NOTES: To increase the dosage
of THC, you can add a small amount of
cannabis ghee to the skillet when you cook
the grilled cheese. For each 1 teaspoon
ghee you add, you will be adding about
17.5 mg per sandwich.

Serve the sandwiches with chilled Tomato
Gazpacho (page 101).

1 In a bowl, whisk together the mayonnaise and mustard. Set aside.

2 In another bowl, mix together the thyme, rosemary, oregano, and basil. Spread out into an even layer on a sheet pan.

3 Spread a thin skim of the mayonnaise/Dijon mustard mixture on one side of each slice of bread. Flip the slices over and, dividing evenly, spread the Camembert over 4 of the slices.

4 To the remaining mayonnaise/Dijon mustard mixture, add the cannabis ghee and mix until thoroughly incorporated. Add the black pepper, Gruyère, and cheddar to the mixture.

5 Divide the cheese mixture into 4 equal portions. Evenly spread a portion of the cheese blend onto the 4 slices of bread that are bare.

6 Top each with 2 slices of tomato and sandwich together, ensuring that the mayonnaise mixture is on the outside of all 8 slices of bread.

7 Dip the sandwiches on both sides into the mixed herb mixture.

8 Heat a skillet over medium-low heat (see Notes). Add the sandwiches and toast until golden brown and the cheese is melted.

BROKEN

I could always drive down to the Broken Spoke in Austin where the owners, James and Annetta White, treated me like family. They booked me into their beer parlor/dance hall when I was sporting a crew cut and then a lifetime later when my hair was down to my waist. They didn't care. The fans didn't care. It was always home to me. If the walls of the Broken Spoke could speak, they'd talk about the legends who'd played there: Bob Wills, Ernest Tubb, Roy Acuff, Tex Ritter, Ray Price.

I loved the place, not only for its history and music-loving patrons, but its chicken-fried steak. In Texas, chicken-fried steak is a staple, but the Broken Spoke took it to another level. Up there on the bandstand toward the end of a set, I was conflicted. The fans kept calling out for more songs—and I'm a guy who always wants to please his fans—but at the same time I was hungry as a bear. I wanted to sing, but, even more, I wanted to tear into that chicken-fried steak.

There's been a lot of chicken-fried steak in my life, but maybe the best of the best was in Vegas where Benny Binion, the notorious owner of the Horseshoe, invited me and Annie into his private kitchen. That was Annie's first taste of chicken-fried steak—and she loved it.

Try this one Chef Andrea created with a mushroom sauce.

SPOKE

CHICKEN-FRIED STEAK

WITH MUSHROOM SAUCE

MAKES **6 SERVINGS**
17.6 MG PER SERVING

2½ cups all-purpose flour

1 teaspoon smoked paprika

1 teaspoon onion powder

1 teaspoon garlic powder

1 teaspoon baking soda

1 teaspoon baking powder

Kosher salt and freshly ground black pepper

2½ cups buttermilk

3 teaspoons Tabasco sauce

3 large eggs

6 cube steaks (about 5 ounces each)

Vegetable oil, for shallow-frying

MUSHROOM SAUCE

1½ tablespoons unsalted butter

1½ teaspoons Cannabis Ghee (page 9)

1 medium onion, finely chopped

4 garlic cloves, minced

10 ounces mushrooms, sliced

Kosher salt and freshly ground black pepper

Cayenne pepper

½ cup dry white wine

½ cup vegetable broth

½ cup heavy cream

2 teaspoons fresh thyme leaves, chopped

Fresh parsley, chopped, for garnish

1 In a bowl, whisk together the flour, smoked paprika, onion powder, garlic powder, baking soda, baking powder, 1 teaspoon salt, and 1 teaspoon pepper. Set aside.

2 In a separate bowl, whisk together the buttermilk, Tabasco sauce, and eggs. Set aside.

3 Pat the cube steaks dry with a paper towel, removing as much moisture as possible. Season with kosher salt and pepper. Allow them to sit for 5 minutes and pat dry a second time.

4 Dredge the cube steaks in the flour mixture, shaking off the excess, then dredge in the buttermilk/egg mixture, allowing any excess to drip off. Dredge again in the flour mixture while pressing it into the steaks to assure that they are thoroughly coated. Shake off any excess.

5 Place the breaded cube steaks on a sheet pan lined with parchment paper and allow them to sit for 10 minutes.

6 Preheat the oven to 250°F.

7 Meanwhile, line another sheet pan with paper towels and have at the ready. Pour ¼ inch of vegetable oil into a large cast-iron skillet and heat over medium-high heat to 340°F or until oil is hot.

8 Once the oil is up to temperature, place 2 steaks into the pan at a time, and fry until golden brown, 3 to 4 minutes on each side. Remove steaks from pan and drain on paper towels. Place in the preheated oven to keep warm while you make the mushroom sauce.

9 Meanwhile, in a cast-iron or other nonstick skillet, melt the butter and cannabis ghee over medium-high heat. Add the onion and garlic and cook until translucent.

10 Add the mushrooms and season with salt, black pepper, and cayenne pepper to taste. Reduce the heat to medium and cook until the mushrooms reduce in size and are golden brown.

11 Add the wine and cook until the liquids are reduced by half. Add the vegetable broth and simmer until the liquids have reduced by half, about 5 minutes.

12 Add the heavy cream and fresh thyme and cook, stirring occasionally, until the sauce thickens enough to coat the back of a spoon, 3 to 5 minutes. Remove from the heat.

13 To serve, set a chicken-fried steak on each of six plates. Divide the mushroom sauce evenly over the steaks. Garnish with the chopped parsley.

VEGAN BEER-BATTERED FISH SANDWICHES

MAKES **8 SANDWICHES**   **13.25 MG** PER SERVING
(ADD **5.85 MG** PER SERVING IF USING VEGAN DILL & CAVIAR TARTAR SAUCE)
(ADD **17.6 MG** PER SERVING IF USING VEGAN HEMP HEART BUNS)

VEGAN "FISH" PATTIES

1½ teaspoons Vegan Cannabis Butter (page 9)

1 tablespoon neutral oil, plus more for the baking dish

1 tablespoon minced garlic

18 ounces canned banana blossom, drained and roughly chopped

18 ounces canned hearts of palm, drained and diced

2 tablespoon kelp granules or dulse flakes

1 tablespoon vegan fish sauce

1 tablespoon garlic powder

1½ teaspoons onion powder

¼ cup chickpea flour

1 cup panko bread crumbs

Kosher salt

FOR BATTER-FRYING

1 quart oil, for frying

2 cups all-purpose flour

½ teaspoon baking powder

1 tablespoon garlic powder

1 tablespoon sweet paprika

1 teaspoon lemon-pepper seasoning

Pinch kosher salt

1½ cups beer

FOR SERVING

8 Vegan Hemp Heart Buns (optional; page 234)

Vegan Dill and Caviar Tartar Sauce (optional; recipe follows)

Tomatoes

Lettuce

Vegan cheese

---

1 In a skillet, combine the vegan cannabis butter and neutral oil and heat over medium heat. Add the minced garlic and cook until aromatic.

2 Add the roughly chopped banana blossom and sauté for 2 to 3 minutes.

3 Add the hearts of palm, kelp granules, fish sauce, garlic powder, and onion powder. Cook until the combination is warmed through. Remove from the heat and allow it to cool completely.

4 Meanwhile, in a small bowl, whisk enough water into the chickpea flour until it reaches the consistency of beaten eggs.

continues

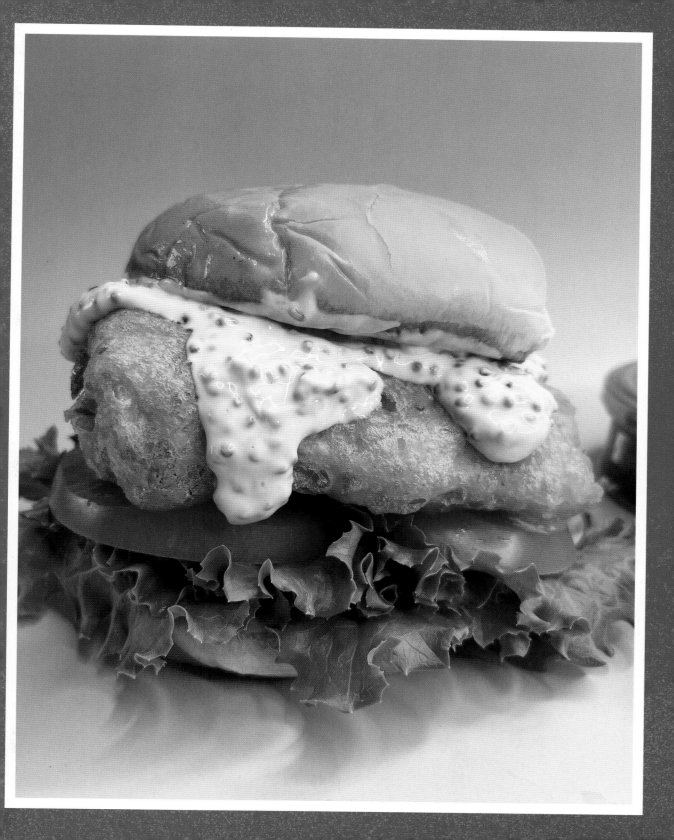

VEGAN BEER-BATTERED FISH SANDWICHES

continued

5 Once the "fish" mixture is cool, season with kosher salt to taste. (Slightly oversalt the mixture because adding the next ingredients may diminish the flavor.) Add the chickpea mixture and gently fold until well combined. Add the panko and repeat. Refrigerate for 30 minutes to allow the mixture to set .

6 Preheat the oven to 350°F. Lightly oil an 8 x 25-inch baking dish.

7 Remove the mixture from the refrigerator and divide into 8 equal portions and roll into balls. Form the balls into square patties similar to Filet-O-Fish and place in the oiled baking dish in single layer.

8 Bake until the patties are slightly firm, 30 to 45 minutes.

9 Remove from the oven and let the patties cool completely. Refrigerate for 20 minutes.

10 Set up a wire rack in a sheet pan and have near the stove. Pour the oil into a deep heavy pot or deep-fryer and heat to 340°F on a deep-fry thermometer.

11 Meanwhile, in a bowl, whisk together the flour, baking powder, garlic powder, paprika, lemon-pepper seasoning, and salt until well combined. Slowly whisk in the beer until the consistency of the batter is smooth.

12 Working in batches (to not crowd the pan), with impeccably clean or gloved hands, coat the "fish" patties in the beer batter and place gingerly into the hot oil. Fry until golden brown. Remove from the oil and drain on the wire rack. Repeat with the remaining patties.

13 If desired, serve on a hemp heart bun with 1½ tablespoons tartar sauce and any preferred toppings.

VEGAN DILL & CAVIAR TARTAR SAUCE

MAKES ¾ **CUP** (12 TABLESPOONS)
11.7 MG PER SERVING (3 TABLESPOONS)

½ cup vegan
   mayonnaise
1 tablespoon finely
   diced shallots
1 teaspoon fresh
   lemon juice
1 teaspoon garlic
   powder
1 teaspoon Cannabis
   Grapeseed Oil
   (page 11)

2 tablespoons Zeroe
   Caviar (or other
   brand of vegan
   caviar)
1 teaspoon chopped
   fresh dill

In a small bowl, whisk together the mayonnaise, shallots, lemon juice, garlic powder, and cannabis oil. Gently fold in the vegan caviar and dill until well incorporated. Refrigerate for an hour before serving.

HOME FOR

HO

THE
OLIDAYS

SONGS

Vegetables as well as meat can be tainted with pesticides and poisons. Organic and regenerative farmers are a gift and we should recognize and support them. Farming, like music, is magical. Songs and soil are rooted in mystery. Both require loving cultivation.

I've lived the farm life. I love the tastes and smells.

I've been shaped by the farm life. As a kid, that's all I knew. It grounded me. I learned the satisfaction of cultivating the land in a way that the land allows you to live.

Pickin' food in the fields. Pickin' on my guitar. Getting to the right rhythms. The natural rhythms. Staying in tune with the mystical forces that feed our souls.

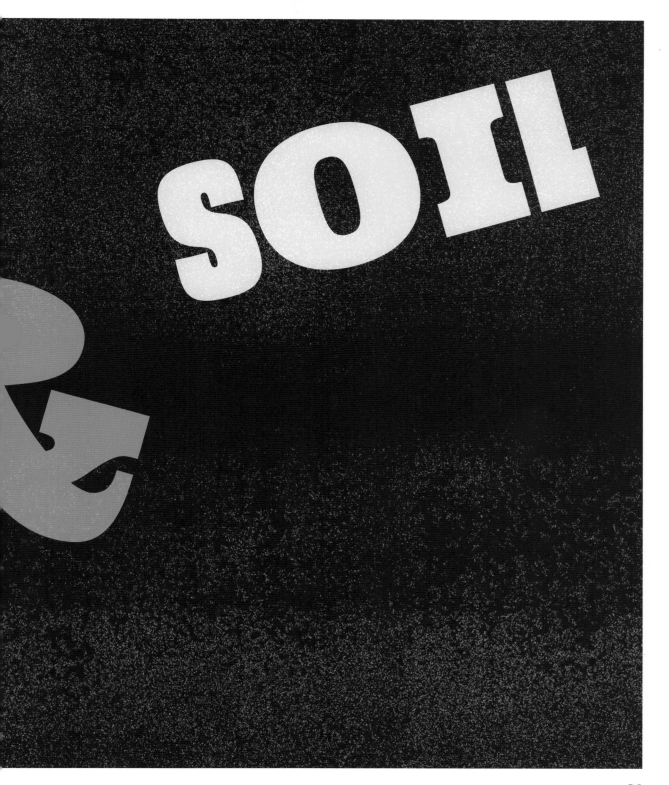

SIMPLE & EASY

Simple and easy suits my style.

That's why I love bananas.

My favorite are the tiny ice cream bananas that grow on Maui.

Bananas are good for you.

Bananas are always available.

I like them straight; I like them in protein shakes; on toast with peanut butter; on ice cream sundaes; fried with butter and brown sugar (and maybe a splash of bourbon).

How about banana bread?

Banana pancakes, banana cream pie, and, best of all, banana pudding.

Which brings me to the good news:

an original recipe for something I find irresistible—*roasted* banana pudding.

ROASTED BANANA PUDDING

MAKES **8 SERVINGS**
26 MG PER SERVING

BANANA CURD
2 large bananas, unpeeled

4 tablespoons unsalted butter, at room temperature

¾ cup packed light brown sugar

Pinch of salt

2 tablespoons Cannabis Ghee (page 9)

2 large eggs

4 large egg yolks

2 tablespoons brandy

½ teaspoon ground cardamom

WHIPPED CREAM
2 cups heavy cream, chilled

2 tablespoons granulated sugar

½ teaspoon vanilla bean paste

ASSEMBLY
8 ounces shortbread cookies, crushed

4 ounces chocolate, shaved

1 ROAST THE BANANAS: Preheat oven to 400°F.

2 Slit the bananas lengthwise through the skin along the top almost all the way to the ends so they stay intact.

3 Place on a baking sheet and roast until the insides of the bananas are soft and starting to bubble, about 15 minutes.

4 MEANWHILE, FOR THE CURD: In a medium bowl, beat the butter, brown sugar, and salt until smooth. Add the cannabis ghee. Add the whole eggs and egg yolks, one at a time, beating until combined before adding the next.

5 When the bananas are cool enough to handle, mash them and measure out ¼ cup plus 2 tablespoons. (Save any roasted banana left over to snack on, maybe with chocolate sauce!) Mix in the roasted banana a little bit at a time. The mixture may separate a little at this point and that is fine.

6 Transfer the mixture to a small pot set over medium-low heat and cook, stirring regularly, until the mixture reaches 175°F on a candy thermometer, about 20 minutes. It should be bubbling periodically, but not at a fast-paced boil.

7 Remove from the heat and transfer to a blender. Add the brandy and cardamom and blend until smooth. Press plastic wrap directly onto the surface of the curd and poke a few holes in it to let the steam release. Refrigerate until ready to use.

8 In a separate bowl, with an electric mixer, beat the heavy cream, granulated sugar, and vanilla bean paste together on high speed until soft peaks form. Chill until ready to assemble.

9 **TO ASSEMBLE:** Layer banana curd, crushed shortbread cookies, and then whipped cream into eight 6-ounce glasses or ramekins. Repeat the layering process and finish with shaved chocolate.

ALL DAY SINGING & DINNER ON THE GROUND

Have you ever had a fried pie after an all-day singing and dinner on the ground church meet? At my first public appearance at age six, I may have been a little nervous. I was wearing a clean white sailor suit and started pickin' my nose. Well, some woman I didn't know was looking at me, and I came out with, "What are you lookin' at me for? I ain't got nothin' to say. If you don't like the looks of me, you can look the other way."

The reward at the end of the day that made everything better was a warm, crispy fried apple pie.

Here's Andrea's take on a fried apple pie.

FRIED APPLE PIES

MAKES **10 PIES**
30.6 MG PER SERVING

PIE DOUGH
3 cups all-purpose flour

2 tablespoons granulated sugar

1 teaspoon fine sea salt

7 tablespoons unsalted butter, cubed

½ cup vegetable shortening

1 tablespoon Cannabis Ghee (page 9)

1 teaspoon apple cider vinegar

6 tablespoons ice water

APPLE FILLING
2 teaspoons Cannabis Avocado Oil (page 10) or Cannabis Grapeseed Oil (page 11)

1¼ cups peeled and cubed Gala apples

1½ cups peeled cubed Granny Smith apples

¼ cup granulated sugar

¼ cup packed dark brown sugar

Grated zest of 1 lemon

2 teaspoons fresh lemon juice

½ teaspoon ground korintje cinnamon

¼ teaspoon kosher salt

1½ teaspoons cornstarch

ASSEMBLY
Egg wash: 1 egg beaten with 1 teaspoon water and a pinch of salt

Neutral oil, for deep-frying

Cinnamon sugar: mix 1 cup of sugar with ¼ cup cinnamon

1 MAKE THE PIE DOUGH: In a large bowl, combine the flour, granulated sugar, and salt. Add the cubed butter, shortening, and cannabis ghee. Cover and chill in the freezer until the ingredients are cold.

2 Using two forks, cut the cold butter and shortening into the flour mixture until it resembles coarse, pebbled sand. Add the vinegar and ice water. Fold to combine until the dough is shaggy.

3 Place the dough on a lightly floured surface and knead until the dough comes together. Form into a square ½ inch thick, cover with plastic wrap, and refrigerate for a minimum of 2 hours or overnight.

4 MAKE THE APPLE FILLING: In a small pot, heat the cannabis oil over medium heat. Add the diced apples, granulated sugar, brown sugar, lemon zest, lemon juice, cinnamon, and salt. Cook over medium heat and stir often until the sugar has dissolved and the apples have softened. Stir in the cornstarch and boil for about 1 minute. The consistency and softness of the apples will differ. That's okay and lends to the texture of the final product. Remove from the heat and allow to cool. Transfer to an airtight container and refrigerate.

5 When ready to make the hand pies, allow the dough to rest at room temperature for 5 minutes.

6 Divide the dough into 4 equal portions. On a lightly floured surface, roll each portion to ¼ inch thick. Cut out as many 4 × 2½-inch rectangles as you can. Repeat rolling out the dough with the remaining 3 portions. Your dough should easily yield 20 rectangles with scraps to spare.

continues

FRIED
APPLE PIES
continued

7 **TO ASSEMBLE:** Use a pastry brush to apply the egg wash to the perimeter of all the pie dough rectangles. Spoon 1 tablespoon of the apple filling into the center of each of 10 rectangles. Invert the remaining egg-washed rectangles over filling. Ensure the egg-washed borders are facing each other. Line up the edges of the top and bottom pieces and use a fork to seal the edges together.

8 Place the pies on a parchment-lined baking sheet. Cover and freeze while you heat the frying oil.

9 Set a wire rack in a sheet pan and set near the stove. Pour 4 inches of oil into a Dutch oven or deep-fryer and heat the oil to 365°F on a deep-fry thermometer.

10 Working in batches of 2 to 3 chilled hand pies at a time, being careful not to overcrowd the pot, add to the hot oil and fry until golden brown, 2 to 3 minutes on each side. Drain on a wire rack.

11 Dust with cinnamon sugar and serve. The pies can be served warm or at room temperature.

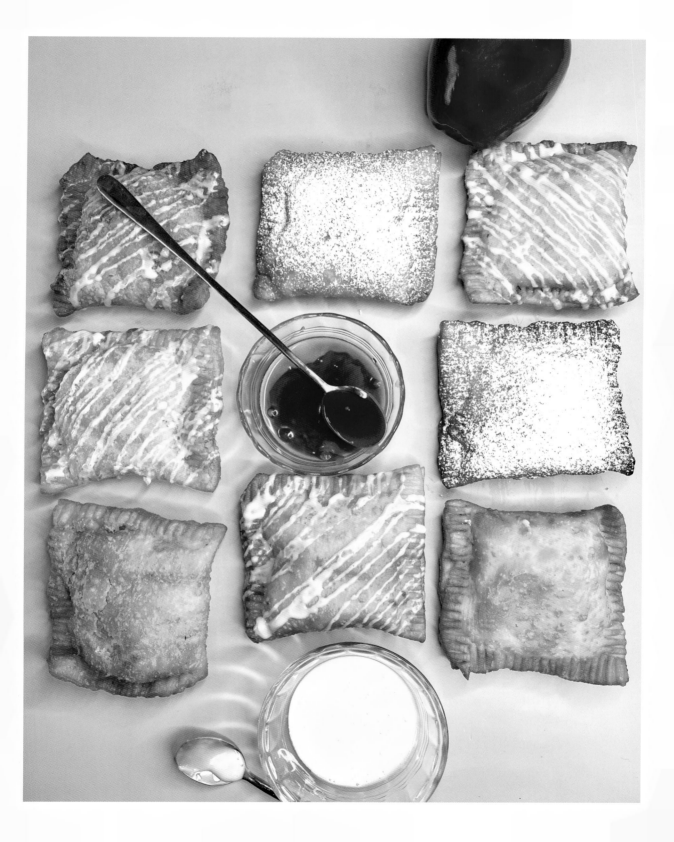

BOURBON PECAN BARS

MAKES **24 BARS**
17.6 MG PER SERVING

DOUGH

1¾ cups all-purpose flour

⅔ cup powdered sugar

¼ cup cornstarch

½ teaspoon kosher salt

12 tablespoons (6 ounces) cold unsalted butter, diced

FILLING

1¼ cups packed light brown sugar

½ cup light corn syrup

2 tablespoons Cannabis Ghee (page 9)

2 teaspoons unsalted butter

2 tablespoons bourbon

4 cups coarsely chopped pecans

½ cup heavy cream

2 teaspoons vanilla bean paste

1 Preheat the oven to 350°F. Line a 9 × 13-inch baking pan with nonstick foil, leaving about 1 inch of overhang.

2 MAKE THE DOUGH: In a food processor, mix together the flour, powdered sugar, cornstarch, and salt. Add the butter and process until the mixture clumps together.

3 Pour into the baking pan and press evenly. Bake for 20 minutes or until golden brown. Cook time may vary according to altitude. Remove and set aside.

4 Reduce the oven temperature to 325°F.

5 MEANWHILE, MAKE THE FILLING: In a medium saucepan, combine the brown sugar, corn syrup, cannabis ghee, unsalted butter, and bourbon and stir over medium-high heat until the sugar dissolves and the mixture boils.

6 Add the pecans and cream and boil until it thickens slightly. Stir in the vanilla bean paste.

7 Pour the filling over the baked crust and return to the oven. Bake until the caramel darkens and bubbles.

8 Transfer to a rack to cool completely before cutting into 24 bars.

SQUID INK PAELLA

MAKES **6 SERVINGS**
23.5 MG PER SERVING

2 tablespoons olive oil

½ pound squid, cleaned and sliced into ¼-inch rings

1½ tablespoons ground crayfish

1 tablespoon Cajun boudin seasoning

1 yellow onion, finely diced

1 red bell pepper, diced

1 tablespoon Cannabis Avocado Oil (page 10)

4 garlic cloves, minced

2 teaspoons smoked paprika

1 teaspoon ground cumin

2 pinches of saffron threads

2 tablespoons tomato paste

1 tablespoon crab paste

1½ cups bomba rice or Arborio rice

1 cup dry white wine

4¼ cups seafood or vegetable stock

¼ cup squid ink

1½ cups cherry tomatoes

1 pound shell-on prawns

Lemon wedges, for serving

Chopped fresh parsley, for garnish

1 Preheat the oven to 350°F.

2 In a paella pan or wide skillet, heat the olive oil over medium heat. Once the oil is up to temperature, add the squid rings and sauté for 30 seconds. Remove from the pan and set aside.

3 Add the ground crayfish and boudin seasoning and toast the seasonings for 30 seconds.

4 Add the onion, bell pepper, and cannabis oil and sauté until the onion is soft and translucent, 4 to 5 minutes.

5 Add the garlic, smoked paprika, cumin, and saffron and sauté until aromatic. Stir in the tomato paste and crab paste and cook for another 2 minutes.

6 Add the rice and stir, fully coating the rice with the paste and seasonings. Add the white wine and allow it to simmer for 5 minutes. Add the stock and squid ink and stir until well combined. Adjust the seasoning if needed.

7 Bring the paella to a boil and immediately reduce to a gentle simmer. Without stirring, allow it to simmer until the stock has reduced and the rice is almost cooked.

8 Meanwhile, arrange the cherry tomatoes on a sheet pan, slide into the oven, and roast until they blister but are not burst.

9 Add the prawns on top of the rice and simmer until the rice is fully cooked, 4 to 6 minutes.

10 Add the squid and roasted tomatoes. Remove the paella from the heat and allow it to rest for several minutes.

11 Garnish with lemon wedges and chopped parsley. Serve from the pan.

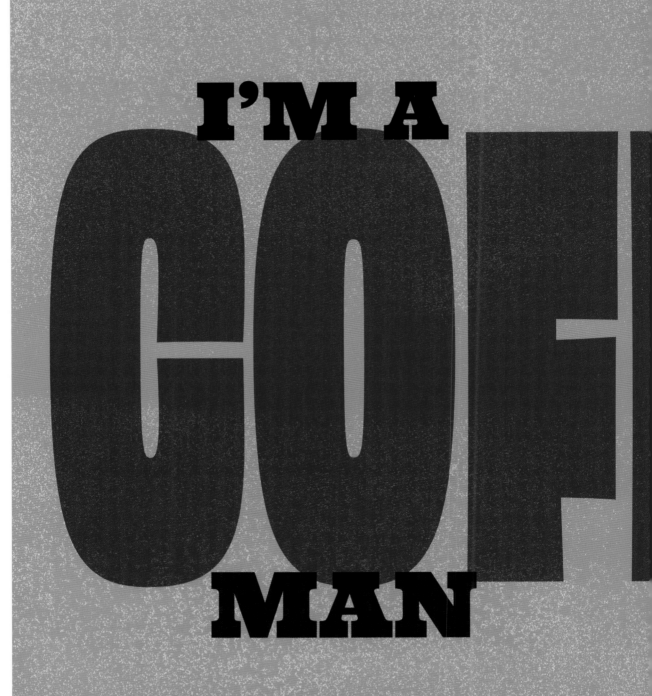

I'M A COFFEE MAN

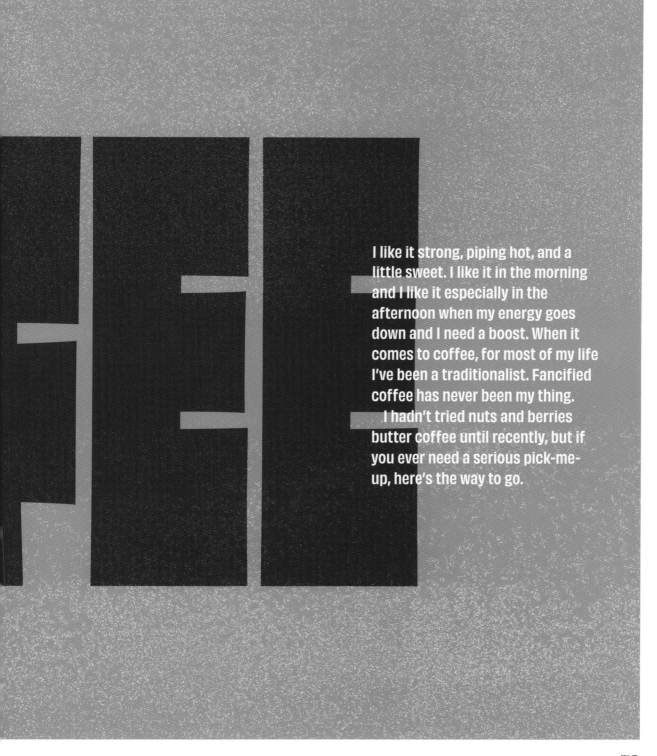

I like it strong, piping hot, and a little sweet. I like it in the morning and I like it especially in the afternoon when my energy goes down and I need a boost. When it comes to coffee, for most of my life I've been a traditionalist. Fancified coffee has never been my thing. I hadn't tried nuts and berries butter coffee until recently, but if you ever need a serious pick-me-up, here's the way to go.

NUTS & BERRIES BUTTER COFFEE

MAKES **2 SERVINGS**
17.6 MG PER SERVING
(ADD **1.4 MG** PER SERVING IF USING
VANILLA BEAN WHIPPED CREAM)

2 cups brewed black cold coffee

2 tablespoons butter

½ teaspoon Cannabis Ghee (page 9)

3 tablespoons hazelnut coffee syrup

1 tablespoon raspberry coffee syrup

¼ cup Vanilla Bean Whipped Cream (optional; below)

Hazelnut (optional), for grating

1 In a blender, combine the cold coffee, butter, cannabis ghee, hazelnut coffee syrup, and raspberry coffee syrup and blend on high speed until the mixture is well combined and frothed.

2 Divide between two cups. If using the whipped cream, dollop 2 tablespoons onto each coffee. Using a Microplane grater, garnish the whipped cream with grated hazelnut.

VANILLA BEAN WHIPPED CREAM

MAKES **2 CUPS** (32 TABLESPOONS)
1.4 MG PER SERVING (2 TABLESPOONS)

1 cup heavy whipping cream

1 teaspoon vanilla bean paste

¼ cup Cannabis-Infused Simple Syrup (page 213)

In a bowl, with an electric mixer, beat the cream, vanilla bean paste, and infused simple syrup until soft peaks form. Refrigerate until ready to use.

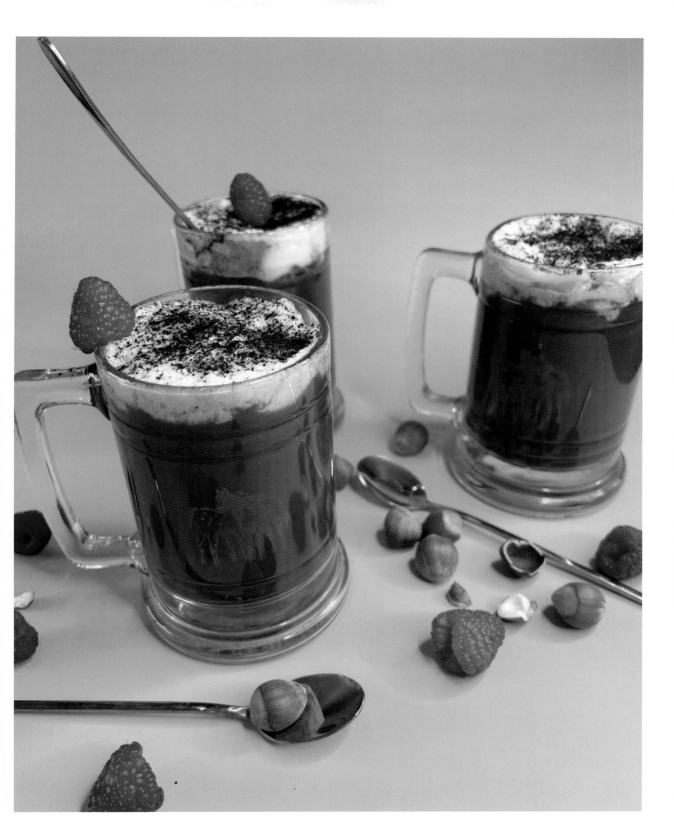

When we are home in Maui, Annie can get the freshest foods on our table every day. It's an opportunity to recharge my energy and boost my health. Every so often my buddy Woody Harrelson goes on a juice cleanse. He calls it a "clean up" and sometimes I join in. That's where the fresh veggies come in. But my approach is different than his. You see, after a few days, a juice cleanse can make a fella a little foggy in the head. So on day three or four, I stop while Woody keeps it going.

That usually brings us to the poker table. For all his brilliance as an actor, Woody can forget that, during the deep days of his "clean up," his powers of concentration can be compromised.

Do I take advantage of that? Well, poker—at least the way we play it—might best be described as cutthroat. That means that sometimes during one of Woody's juice cleanses, I'm the one who cleans up.

Here's a recipe for a drink with lots of juice in it. It was inspired by the beat poet Allen Ginsberg who said, "There is not beat poetry, or a beat novel, or beat painting. Beat is a poetic conception, an attitude toward the world."

JUICE CLEANSE

BEET NICK COCKTAIL

MAKES **1 COCKTAIL**
8 MG PER DRINK

**2 ounces MXXN Kentucky
    Oak cannabis-infused
    nonalcoholic spirit**

4 ounces beet juice

1 tablespoon ginger juice

1 tablespoon honey

Squeeze of lemon

Ice or Collins ice

Lemon peel, for garnish

In a cocktail mixing glass, combine the infused spirit, beet juice, ginger juice, honey, and lemon juice. Using a small bar whisk, blend until well combined. Pour into an 8-ounce Collins glass over mixing ice cubes or Collins ice. Stir with a bar spoon. Garnish with lemon peel and serve.

CHRISTMAS MEANS MEMORIES

One of my favorite memories is Christmas dinner in Montreux. It was 1984. I was with Johnny Cash, Waylon Jennings, and Kris Kristofferson. All of us had brought our families.

Johnny had flown us over to Europe for one of his shows. On Christmas Day we all wound up in a wonderful little restaurant in the middle of the Alps. We ate on picnic tables outside where the air was clean, the sky clear. Yodelers and folk dancers added to the idyllic setting.

Most beautiful of all was the fellowship between my friends and our families. This led to the formation of a group we called the Highwaymen. (Kris characterized us best: "Willie's the outlaw cowboy, Waylon's the riverboat gambler, I'm the radical, and John is the father of our country.")

That group made records and traveled the world, but nothing we did would ever be as sweet as that Christmas dinner.

Here's a Christmas dinner recipe that I hope brings you good cheer and lots of love.

HOLIDAY LEG OF LAMB WITH MINT GREMOLATA

MAKES **8 SERVINGS**
17.6 MG PER SERVING

4-pound leg of lamb, bone in

1 bulb garlic, chopped

Grated zest and juice of 1 lemon

½ bunch fresh rosemary, chopped

1 cup olive oil

Kosher salt and freshly ground black pepper

MINT GREMOLATA

4 garlic cloves, minced

1 teaspoon grated lemon zest

1 teaspoon fresh lemon juice

2 cups loosely packed fresh mint leaves, finely chopped

½ loosely packed fresh parsley, finely chopped

2 tablespoons olive oil

1 tablespoon Cannabis Grapeseed Oil (page 11)

Kosher salt

CHEF'S NOTE: Serve the lamb with Roasted Hasselback Potatoes (page 80).

1 Trim off extra fat from the lamb and refrigerate it for 2 hours. Remove the lamb from the fridge and allow it to come up to room temperature.

2 Preheat the oven to 400°F.

3 In a bowl, stir together the garlic, lemon zest, lemon juice, rosemary, and olive oil. Season the lamb with salt and pepper, then drizzle with the marinade, thoroughly rubbing it all over the meat. Place on the rack of a roasting pan and cook the leg of lamb to 160°F internal temperature for medium or 170°F for well done, about 1 hour 15 minutes. Cook 15 minutes longer if you prefer less pink. Let rest before carving.

4 MEANWHILE, MAKE THE MINT GREMOLATA: In a bowl, combine the garlic, lemon zest, lemon juice, mint, parsley, olive oil, and cannabis oil. Mix until well combined. Season with kosher salt to taste.

5 To serve, carve in thin slices with a carving knife or slicer. Garnish each serving with 5 tablespoons of the gremolata.

ROASTED HASSELBACK POTATOES

MAKES **8 SERVINGS**
8.8 MG PER SERVING (2 POTATOES)

16 small to medium Yukon Gold potatoes, rinsed and dried

5 tablespoons avocado oil

4 tablespoons unsalted butter, melted

1 teaspoon Cannabis Ghee (page 9)

4 garlic cloves, minced

1 tablespoon chopped fresh rosemary

Sea salt and freshly ground black pepper

CHEF'S NOTE: These are great served warm with Holiday Leg of Lamb with Mint Gremolata (page 79).

1 Preheat the oven to 350°F.

2 Place a chopstick on either side of a potato and cut the potato into slices about ⅛ inch apart, stopping when you hit the chopsticks. Repeat for all the potatoes.

3 Add the potatoes to a bowl and drizzle in the avocado oil. Gently hand toss to evenly distribute the oil.

4 Transfer the potatoes to a 18 x 25-inch baking dish and arrange so that they're snug but not on top of each other. Bake at 350°F until golden and crispy on top, about 1 hour. Let cool for about 2 minutes.

5 In a bowl, stir together the melted butter, cannabis ghee, garlic, and rosemary. Add the potatoes and evenly coat using a mixing spoon or rubber spatula. Season with the sea salt and black pepper.

GLAZED CARROTS

MAKES **8 SERVINGS**
5.8 MG PER SERVING

8 tablespoons vegan butter

4 pounds medium carrots, peeled and halved lengthwise

½ cup packed light brown sugar

1 teaspoon cayenne pepper

1 teaspoon Cannabis Coconut Oil (page 10)

1 teaspoon kosher salt

CHEF'S NOTE: Pair these with Holiday Leg of Lamb (page 79).

1 In a large skillet, melt the vegan butter over medium heat. Add the carrots and cook, stirring occasionally, until tender, 8 to 10 minutes.

2 Stir in the brown sugar, cayenne, and cannabis oil. Cook until the sugar is dissolved and the carrots are coated and slightly caramelized. Season with the salt.

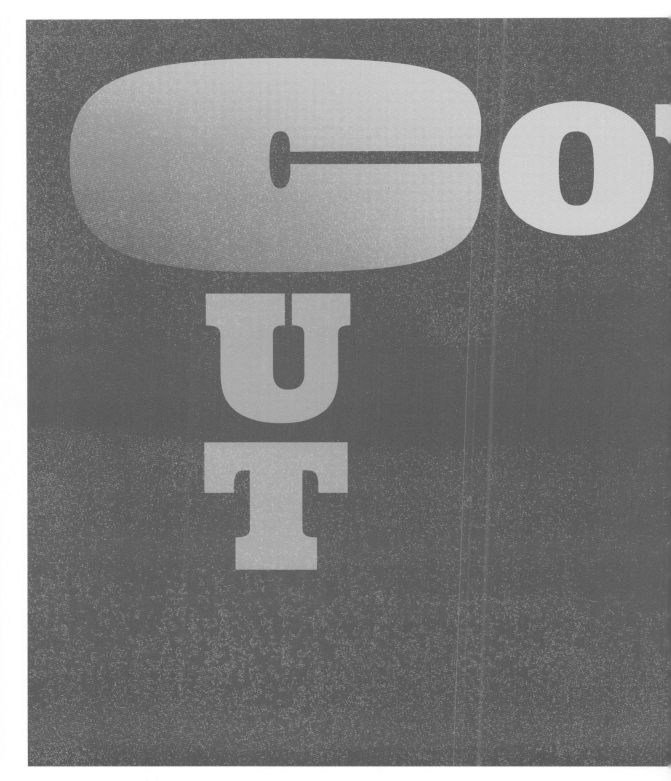

WBOY

Sometimes the farther you roam from home, the closer you get.

I'm thinking about Perth, the capital of Western Australia. It reminded me of home. Vast landscape. Big sky. A sense of openness. Openhearted people who love country music as much as the fans in Austin or Amarillo.

I was over there in the nineties with the Highwaymen. Whether it was Johnny Cash singing "Folsom Prison Blues," Kris Kristofferson singing "Help Me Make It Through the Night," or me and Waylon Jennings singing "Luckenbach Texas (Back to the Basics of Love)," the reception was great.

So was the food. Especially the steaks. They were grass-fed, tender, and full of flavor. Huge steaks cooked over huge grills and served on huge plates.

There are a million and one ways to prepare steaks. I'll always remember the Aussie way, but here's a recipe for a sauce that will make any steak extra-special.

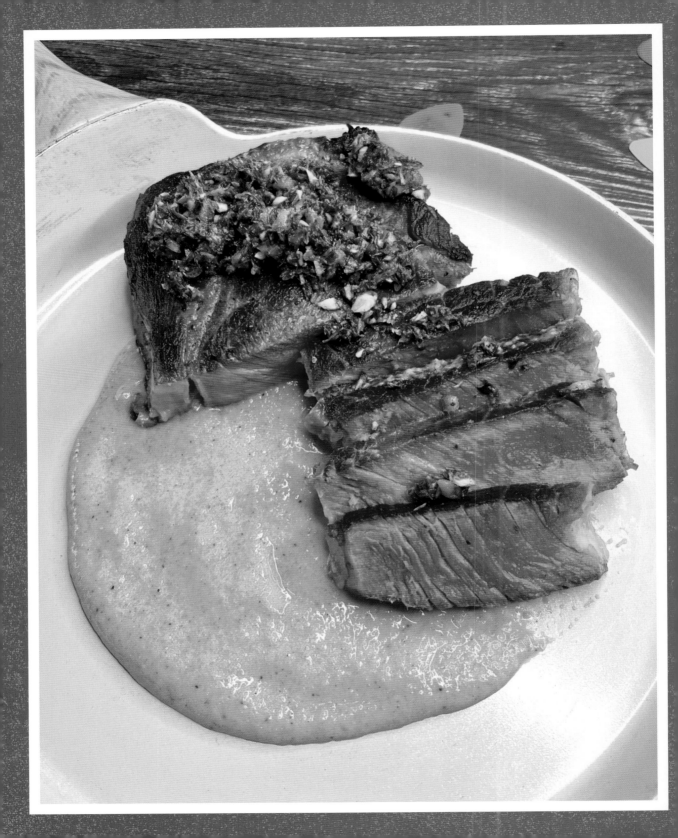

SOUS-VIDE STEAK WITH AJÍ AMARILLO (PERUVIAN YELLOW CHILE)

MAKES **6 SERVINGS**
23.5 MG PER SERVING

AJÍ AMARILLO SAUCE
½ cup mayonnaise

¼ cup Mexican crema

2 tablespoons ají amarillo paste

1 tablespoon tomato paste

1 tablespoon Cannabis Grapeseed Oil (page 11)

2 tablespoons fresh lime juice, plus more to taste

¼ cup crumbled queso fresco

1 small shallot, minced

2 garlic cloves, peeled but whole

Kosher salt and freshly ground black pepper

SOUS-VIDE STEAKS
6 New York strip steaks cut 1 inch thick

Kosher salt and freshly ground black pepper

12 sprigs fresh thyme

3 tablespoons neutral oil, divided

3 tablespoons ghee

1 MAKE THE AJÍ AMARILLO SAUCE: In a food processor or blender, combine the mayo, crema, aji amarillo paste, tomato paste, cannabis oil, lime juice, queso fresco, shallot, and garlic and process until smooth. Adjust the seasoning with salt and pepper to taste. Transfer to a bowl and refrigerate until ready to serve.

2 Meanwhile, preheat a large water bath using an immersion circulator to 129°F for medium-rare steaks, 135°F for medium, or 145°F for well-done.

3 Liberally season the steaks with the salt and pepper.

4 Place 2 sprigs of fresh thyme in each bag along with equal amounts of neutral oil (to equal 2 tablespoons). Individually vacuum-seal the seasoned steaks or use the air removal method with a zip-top plastic bag.

5 Add the sealed steaks to the preheated water bath and make sure they are submerged. Cook for 1 to 3 hours.

continues

SOUS-VIDE STEAK WITH AJÍ AMARILLO (PERUVIAN YELLOW CHILE)

continued

CHEF'S NOTE: Feeling ambitious? Garnish with the mint gremolata from Holiday Leg of Lamb (page 79). This recipe can also be served with Chimichurri Special (page 87).

The air removal method is to remove all the air from the ziplock bag before sealing.

6 Remove the steaks from the water bath and the bags and transfer to a sheet pan. Pat the steaks completely dry with paper towels.

7 Preheat a cast-iron skillet over high heat until the skillet is smoking. Make sure to turn on the vent over your stove. Once smoking, add 1 tablespoon of ghee and melt. Add 2 steaks and sear for about 30 seconds on each side. Be careful to not go too long or you'll risk overcooking the steak. Repeat with more ghee until all the steaks are cooked to perfection.

8 Dividing evenly, pour the aji amarillo sauce on each of six plates. Add the steak.

CHIMICHURRI
SPECIAL

MAKES **4 CUPS** (64 TABLESPOONS)
8.8 MG PER SERVING (2 TABLESPOONS)

1½ cups olive oil

2 tablespoons red wine vinegar

2 tablespoons Cannabis Avocado Oil (page 10) or Cannabis Grapeseed Oil (page 11)

½ cup finely chopped fresh parsley

½ cup finely chopped fresh cilantro

½ cup finely chopped fresh mint

4 garlic cloves, minced

2 Thai chiles, finely chopped

¾ teaspoon dried oregano

2 teaspoons coarse salt

In a bowl, stir together all of the ingredients until well blended. Allow the chimichurri sauce to sit for at least 2 hours so that all of the flavors meld together and infuse the oil.

BIRRIA QUESO DIP

MAKES **8 SERVINGS**
17.6 MG PER SERVING

2 tablespoons neutral oil

1 tablespoon Cannabis Avocado Oil (page 10) or Cannabis Grapeseed Oil (page 11)

1 onion, diced

4 garlic cloves, minced

1 pound braised short rib (see Note), chopped

2½ tablespoons Chile Paste (recipe follows)

1 tablespoon ground cumin

2 teaspoons ground coriander

2 teaspoons smoked paprika

1 teaspoon ground korintje cinnamon

1 teaspoon ground cloves

Kosher salt

1 cup half-and-half

4 cups shredded white American cheese

3 cups shredded mozzarella cheese

Chopped fresh cilantro, for garnish

Finely diced onion, for garnish

Tortilla chips, for serving

1 In a large cast-iron skillet, heat the neutral oil and cannabis oil over medium heat. Add the onion and cook until translucent.

2 Add the garlic and cook for about 1 minute. Add the chopped meat, chile paste, cumin, coriander, smoked paprika, cinnamon, and cloves. Mix thoroughly and cook over low heat until warmed through. Remove from the heat and set aside.

4 In a saucepan, bring the half-and-half to a simmer over medium heat. Whisk in both cheeses in small handfuls until completely melted and the queso is very smooth. This should take about 5 minutes.

5 Scoop the queso into a serving dish and top with the meat mixture. Garnish with cilantro and diced onion. Serve with tortilla chips.

CHEF'S NOTE: You can use any cooked meat or poultry here, but short rib has a deep richness that is perfect for birria-style dishes.

CHILE PASTE

4 dried ancho chiles, seeded and stemmed

4 dried guajillo chiles, seeded and stemmed

3 dried chiles de árbol, seeded and stemmed

1 teaspoon kosher salt

1 In a bowl, combine the chiles with water to cover and let rehydrate for at least 6 hours or overnight.

2 Drain the chiles. In a blender, combine the chiles, salt, and 1 teaspoon water. Blend until smooth, adding more water as needed to achieve a paste-like consistency.

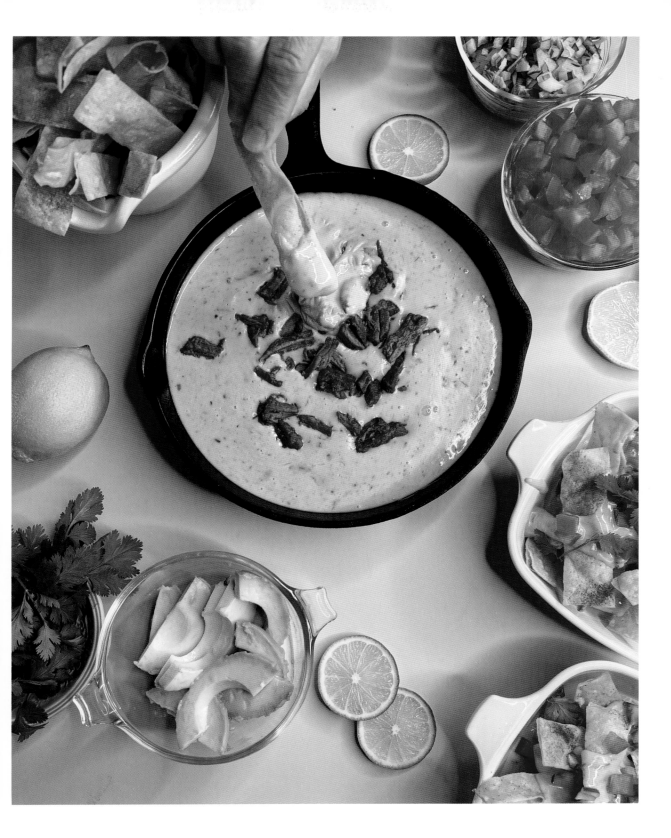

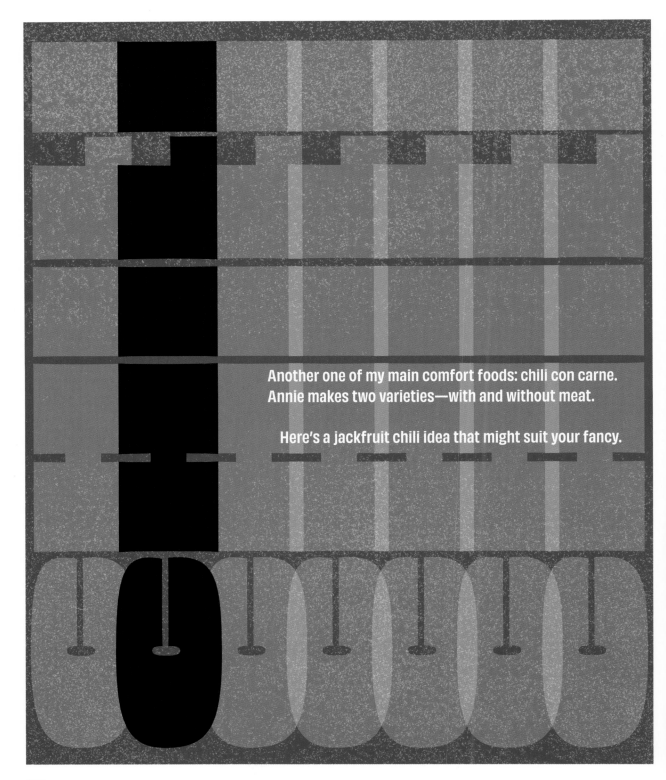

Another one of my main comfort foods: chili con carne.
Annie makes two varieties—with and without meat.

Here's a jackfruit chili idea that might suit your fancy.

JACKFRUIT CHILI

MAKES **8 SERVINGS**
17.6 MG PER SERVING

- 4 (14-ounce) cans young green jackfruit, drained
- 1 cup TVP (textured vegetable protein)
- 2 tablespoons olive oil
- 2 teaspoons Cannabis Avocado Oil (page 10) or Cannabis Grapeseed Oil (page 11)
- 2 cups diced yellow onion
- 1 cup finely diced poblano chile
- 8 garlic cloves, minced
- ⅓ cup ancho chile powder
- 2 tablespoons ground cumin
- 1 tablespoon kosher salt
- 1½ teaspoon black cocoa powder
- 1½ teaspoons ground korintje cinnamon
- 1 teaspoon freshly ground black pepper
- 1 (6-ounce) can tomato paste
- 1 teaspoon fresh thyme leaves
- 1 teaspoon chopped fresh oregano
- 1½ cups dried red kidney beans, soaked overnight and cooked
- 1 cup dried black beans, soaked overnight and cooked
- 3⅓ cups canned diced San Marzano tomatoes
- 3⅓ cups vegetable broth
- Toppings: shredded cheese, jalapeños, radishes, cilantro, onion, avocado, or sour cream

1 Squeeze excess moisture from the drained jackfruit. Break it up into bite-size pieces or shreds. Set aside.

2 In a bowl, submerge the TVP in water to rehydrate it. Set aside.

3 In a large pot, heat the olive oil and cannabis oil over medium-high heat. Add the onion, poblano, and garlic and cook, stirring frequently, until tender.

4 Reduce the heat to medium, add the jackfruit, and cook for 2 to 5 minutes until the jackfruit is tender. Add the TVP and stir for an additional 2 minutes. Stir in the ancho powder, cumin, salt, black cocoa, cinnamon, and black pepper and toast until fragrant.

5 Add the tomato paste and slightly increase the heat. Then add the thyme and oregano, stirring frequently. Add the cooked beans, diced tomatoes, and vegetable broth. Bring the ingredients to a boil. Reduce the heat to medium-low and simmer, stirring occasionally, until cooked through, about 30 minutes.

6 Serve the chili with any or all of your preferred toppings.

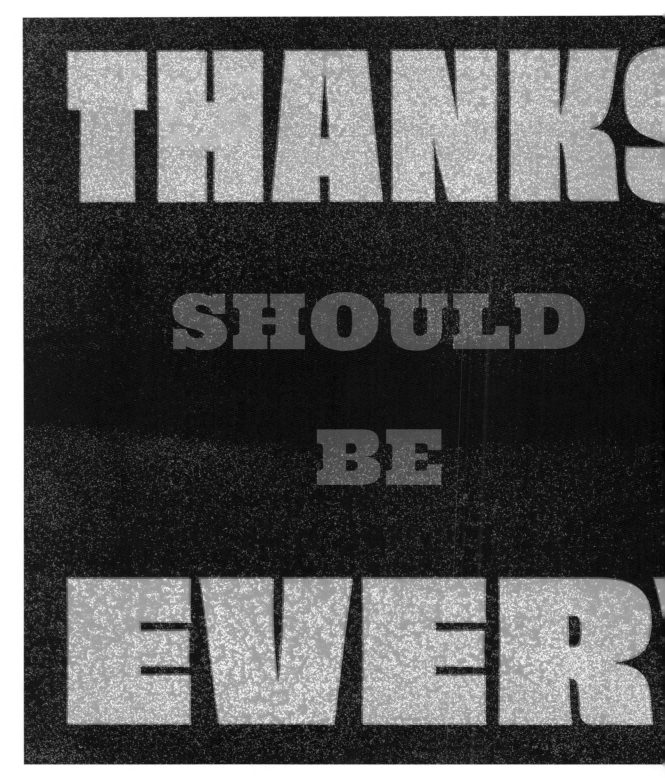

GIVING

Every hour.
   Every minute.
   Every time we take a deep breath.
   Every time we drink a glass of water or eat a piece of bread.
   Gratitude is the gravy of positive thought.
   I try to pour it over everything.
   Sure, it's beautiful to have the ritual of that November day when we sit around the table with our loved ones.
   Feasts are fabulous, and you'll see I'm offering up a Thanksgiving recipe with a twist all its own.
   Enjoy the day. Enjoy the food. Enjoy that warm holiday glow.
   And, as for me, I'll be with you in spirit as I try to stretch this gratitude thing as far as it will go.

Y DAY

ROASTED TURKEY SANDWICHES WITH CRANBERRY AIOLI

MAKES **6 SANDWICHES**
12.7 MG PER SERVING

1 small whole turkey (8 pounds)

2 sticks (8 ounces) unsalted butter, at room temperature

10 sprigs fresh rosemary

10 sprigs fresh thyme

Kosher salt and freshly ground black pepper

½ cup Cannabis-Infused Mayonnaise (page 165)

¾ cup Cannabis-Infused Cranberry Sauce (page 95)

12 slices Tuscan bread, toasted

Sliced tomatoes

Pea shoots

1 Preheat the oven to 325°F.

2 Set the turkey in a roasting pan. Taking care not to puncture the skin, rub half of the softened butter under the skin of the turkey. Then insert the rosemary and thyme sprigs, again being careful not to break the skin. Rub the remaining butter on the outside of the skin and season with kosher salt and black pepper.

3 Transfer the turkey to the oven and roast until the internal temperature of the breast is 165°F, about 2½ hours. Intermittently, baste the turkey with the pan drippings.

4 Remove the turkey from the oven and transfer to a cutting board. Allow it to rest for 30 minutes before carving.

5 Meanwhile, in a bowl, combine the cannabis mayonnaise and infused cranberry sauce. Season with salt to taste and mix until well combined.

6 To build the sandwiches, spread 6 slices of the toasted bread with an equal amount of the cranberry aioli (a scant 3½ tablespoons). Add the sliced turkey, sliced tomato, and pea shoots. Close the lid, slice the sandwiches in half, and serve.

CANNABIS-INFUSED CRANBERRY SAUCE

MAKES **2 CUPS** (32 TABLESPOONS)
8.8 MG PER SERVING (2 TABLESPOONS)

1 (12-ounce) bag cranberries, rinsed

¾ cup packed light brown sugar

3 tablespoons minced fresh ginger

¼ cup fresh orange juice

1 tablespoon grated orange zest

1 tablespoon Cannabis Grapeseed Oil (page 11)

½ teaspoon pure vanilla extract

1 Measure out ½ cup cranberries and set aside (you will stir these in at the end for extra texture).

2 In a medium saucepan, combine the remaining cranberries, ¾ cup water, the brown sugar, ginger, and orange juice. Stir occasionally as the mixture comes to a simmer. Once simmering, reduce the heat to medium-low and continue to cook, stirring occasionally, until the liquid has reduced and the cranberries have burst and thickened.

3 Add the ½ cup cranberries and stir in the orange zest, cannabis oil, and vanilla. Allow the sauce to cool to room temperature. The sauce will continue to thicken as it cools. Store in the refrigerator in an airtight container.

SUPER

>> Lemon Chicken Soup is one of Annie's specialties.

I call it "re-set soup" because it often re-sets our life after months on the road, when we are back home in Hawaii.

The simmering can mean welcome home; it can also mean someone is ailing. It could be the flu; it could be a broken heart; or maybe we're grieving over the passing of a beloved pet.

Whatever the case, that lemon chicken soup is a healing soup—for our family, friends, and neighbors. We have a table that seats twelve, and that table is often full. As our tribe in Maui grows, one thing is sure—no one in our house ever goes hungry.

SOUPS

LEMON CHICKEN SOUP WITH FORBIDDEN RICE

MAKES **6 SERVINGS**
35.3 MG PER SERVING

1 cup Forbidden Rice (black rice)

1 tablespoon Cannabis Avocado Oil (page 10) or Cannabis Grapeseed Oil (page 11)

1 teaspoon Cannabis Ghee (page 9) or Vegan Cannabis Butter (page 9)

½ cup diced yellow onion

½ cup diced peeled carrot

2 celery stalks, diced

4 garlic cloves, minced

2 tablespoons all-purpose flour

6 cups chicken broth

1 pound bone-in, skinless chicken breasts

1 bay leaf

1 tablespoon minced fresh thyme

2 teaspoons minced fresh oregano

1 teaspoon minced fresh rosemary

Grated zest of 1 lemon

2 tablespoons fresh lemon juice

2 tablespoons chopped fresh parsley

Kosher salt and freshly ground black pepper

1 In a pot of boiling water, cook the black rice for 20 minutes to parcook it. Drain and set aside.

2 In a Dutch oven, heat the cannabis oil and cannabis butter over medium heat until melted.

3 Increase the heat to medium-high and immediately add the onion, carrot, and celery. (This prevents the oil and butter from reaching excessive temperatures, which would degrade the THC.) Cook until the onion is translucent, about 5 minutes. Add the garlic and briefly sauté until fragrant.

4 Sprinkle on the flour, stir, and cook until it turns a slightly darker hue than blonde. Deglaze with the chicken broth, stirring/whisking to prevent clumping.

5 Add the whole chicken breasts, bay leaf, and the minced herbs. Bring to a boil. Reduce the heat to a simmer, cover, and cook for 15 minutes.

continues

LEMON CHICKEN SOUP WITH FORBIDDEN RICE

continued

6 Add the parcooked black rice and cook, stirring constantly, for 10 minutes.

7 Remove from the heat. Discard the bay leaf. Remove the chicken and allow it to sit until it has cooled to an internal temperature of 165°F.

8 When the chicken is cool enough to handle, pull the meat off the bones and shred it. Return it to the Dutch oven. Stir in the lemon zest, lemon juice, and parsley.

9 Season with salt and pepper to taste

10 Garnish with sliced lemon rounds and serve.

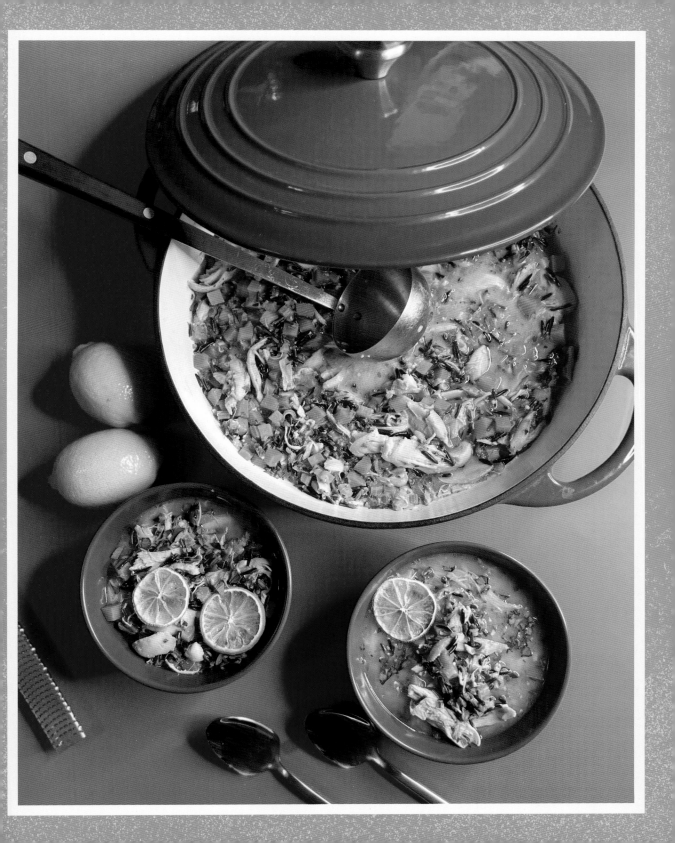

RAW

> **"At least three times each week have almost a full meal of raw vegetables. These should be included at various times; carrots grated, chopped or cut, lettuce, celery, and especially watercress."**
> —EDGAR CAYCE

I was happy to recently stumble across this quote, because during the winter of 1971, when I'd moved back to Texas after a long spell in Tennessee, I started reading Cayce. He was a mystic and a healer who wrote about raising your consciousness. He was also all about deep relaxation. Father A.A. Taliaferro, who married Annie and me in his Dallas office, also had an inspiring take on spirituality that left its mark on me.

All these guys dealt with life's contradictions and how to handle them. How to tolerate and try to understand all the different parts of ourselves. How to live with those parts in harmony rather than have them fighting each other off.

Cooked food is one thing. It's obviously healthy to eat cooked food. At the same time, there's a whole tribe of folks who, like Cayce, remind us that it's also healthy—and even essential—to eat uncooked food. The challenge, then, is how to create raw food meals that are appetizing.

Along those lines, here's an idea . . .

TOMATO GAZPACHO

MAKES **6 SERVINGS**
5.83 MG PER SERVING

1 small red onion

2 pounds heirloom tomatoes, cored and cut into 2-inch chunks

1 cucumber, peeled, seeded, and cut into 2-inch chunks

1 cup chopped red bell pepper

1 cup cubed sourdough bread

¼ cup olive oil

¼ teaspoon Cannabis Avocado Oil (page 10) or Cannabis Grapeseed Oil (page 11)

¼ cup vegetable broth, plus more if needed

¼ cup fresh lime juice, plus more for serving

2 tablespoons chopped, seeded jalapeño

2 garlic cloves

2 tablespoons apple cider vinegar

1 teaspoon salt, plus more to taste

Black pepper to taste

1 teaspoon ground cumin

1 teaspoon ground coriander

2 tablespoons chopped fresh cilantro

1 Fill a bowl with water and ice. Cut the onion into rough 2-inch chunks and let them sit in the ice water for 5 seconds. Drain.

2 In a blender, combine the onion, tomatoes, cucumber, bell pepper, bread, olive oil, cannabis oil, vegetable broth, lime juice, jalapeño, garlic, vinegar, salt, black pepper, ½ teaspoon of the cumin, and ½ teaspoon of the coriander and process until smooth. Season with additional salt and black pepper to taste.

3 Transfer to an airtight container and refrigerate for at least 1 hour and up to 12 hours.

4 To serve, remove the gazpacho from the refrigerator and thin with additional vegetable broth if needed to reach the desired consistency. Garnish with the cilantro and additional lime juice, and remaining ½ teaspoon of the cumin and coriander each.

CHEF'S NOTE: This pairs well with Herb-Crusted Grilled Cheese (page 50); 10.4 mg per serving.

CAN A MEAL TELL A STORY?

WHY NOT?

Songs tell stories, even those without lyrics.

For decades, I've been playing a wordless instrumental version of "Nuages," a haunting melody by one of my heroes, the Romanian gypsy guitar genius Django Reinhardt. Every time I do it, a different story line runs through my head: Sometimes it's a lament for a lost lover; sometimes it's a leisurely walk through the French countryside.

A meal featuring fried chicken could tell the story of how I saved my nickels and dimes when I was scratching to make a living in Houston and came home with enough money for my wife, Martha, to cook up a delectable poultry dish for me and our kids, Lana, Susie, and Billy.

Fried chicken could also tell a story about me playing big ol' outdoor picnics where, for the first time, I saw Blacks and Whites partying together. Those stories warm my heart.

At dinner with Oprah in Maui, she called chicken "the soul bird."

I like that. The soul bird has a million stories, and each with a taste of its own. A meal is a love story, from the cook to the people eating. From a mother to child, from man to wife, cooking is love.

VEGAN FRIED CHICKEN SANDWICHES & HOT HONEY

MAKES **6 SERVINGS**
11.7 MG PER SERVING
(ADD **17.6 MG** PER SERVING IF HAVING
ON VEGAN HEMP HEART BUNS)

SEASONED DREDGE

3 cups rice flour

2½ cups all-purpose flour

2 tablespoons smoked paprika

2 tablespoons garlic powder

2 tablespoons onion powder

1 tablespoon Cajun seasoning

1 tablespoon dried oregano

1 tablespoon dried thyme

1 teaspoon adobo seasoning

1 teaspoon freshly ground black pepper

WET BATTER

2 cups unsweetened nondairy milk

2 tablespoons apple cider vinegar

2 tablespoons Cajun seasoning

2 teaspoons garlic powder

2 teaspoons sweet paprika

VEGAN FRIED CHICKEN

1 teaspoon Vegan Cannabis Butter (page 9)

5 teaspoons vegan butter

24 ounces oyster mushrooms

1 quart cooking oil

Vegan Hot Honey (recipe follows)

Red pepper flakes, for sprinkling

6 store-bought vegan sandwich buns or Vegan Hemp Heart Buns (page 234)

Pickles, slaw, tomato slices, lettuce leaves for topping

1 MAKE THE SEASONED DREDGE: In a large bowl, stir together both flours, the smoked paprika, garlic powder, onion powder, Cajun seasoning, oregano, thyme, adobo seasoning, and black pepper. Set aside.

2 MAKE THE WET BATTER: In a separate bowl, mix together the milk, vinegar, Cajun seasoning, garlic powder, and paprika. Set aside.

3 PREPARE THE VEGAN FRIED CHICKEN: In a small bowl, combine the cannabis butter and vegan butter and set aside.

4 Using a wet paper towel, clean the oyster mushrooms. If needed, separate them to make semi-uniform pieces.

5 Set up a large bowl of ice and water. Bring a large pot of water to a boil over medium-high heat. In batches, boil the mushrooms until they are slightly supple yet with a little chew, 2 to 4 minutes. Scoop the mushrooms from the boiling water and transfer to the ice bath. DO NOT allow the mushrooms to linger in the ice bath. Transfer to paper towels and pat dry.

6 Line a wire rack with paper towels and have near the stove. Heat the cooking oil to 370°F in a large pot or use a deep-fryer.

7 Dip the mushrooms into the wet batter mixture and then into the seasoned dredge, pressing the dredge into the mushroom to fully coat.

8 Working in batches, without overcrowding the pot, fry the mushrooms until golden brown, about 3 minutes. Remove with a slotted spoon and transfer to the paper towels. Repeat until all the mushrooms are cooked.

9 Drizzle the chicken-fried mushrooms with hot honey and dust with pepper flakes for added heat.

10 Meanwhile, slice each bun open. Butter each bun with 1 teaspoon of the vegan butter blend. You can use additional vegan butter if needed. In a skillet, toast the open sides of each bun over medium heat.

11 Build the sandwiches using pickles, slaw, tomatoes, and lettuce, and serve hot.

VEGAN HOT HONEY

MAKES **2 CUPS**

2 cups unsweetened
  apple juice
2 cups sugar
¼ cup agave syrup
1 tablespoon fresh
  lemon juice
½ teaspoon orange
  extract
4 to 6 Thai chile
  peppers, slit
  lengthwise

1 In a heavy bottomed medium saucepan, combine the apple juice, sugar, agave syrup, lemon juice, and orange extract. Whisk constantly over medium heat until the sugar dissolves.

2 Add chile peppers according to your heat tolerance. Allow the mixture to come to a rolling boil, stirring occasionally, until bubbles form over the top. Continue to simmer, stirring as needed, for 25 minutes. The color of the mixture will both thicken slightly in texture and darken in color.

3 Remove the honey from the heat and transfer to a heatproof jar. Allow it to cool at room temperature with the lid off. Once cooled, seal and refrigerate overnight.

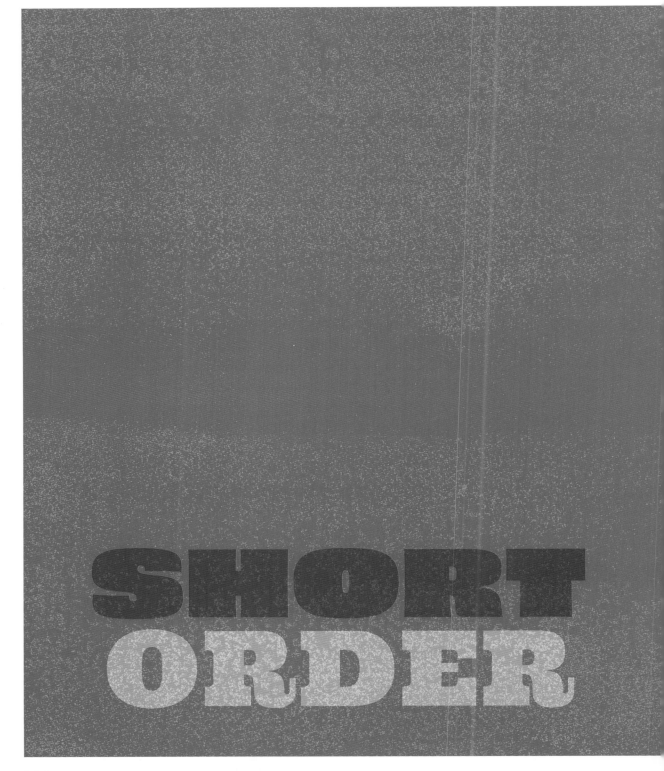

SHORT ORDER

When I keep insisting I'm a simple man, those who know me best push back with "Not as simple as you might think."

This book might be a testament to the truth of their pushback. For instance:

I love watching a good short order cook scrambling eggs with one hand and flipping flapjacks with the other. It's like watching a good drummer. Never misses a beat.

Among Annie's many skills, short-order cooking is one of them. Lukas and Micah always wanted something different to eat— and different from what I was hungering for.

Once, when they were little and we all got home from a long tour, everyone was shouting out orders to Annie.

"This is not a commercial kitchen," she let us all know. "And I am not a short order cook."

We laughed, but the truth is, at the end of the day, she's quicker and better than any short order cook I ever saw. On the bus she'll whip up a couple of eggs over easy with crispy bacon in no time. Along with a cup of strong black coffee.

Simple.

Yet there's nothing simple about Annie's fanciful omelets that she'll create for a dozen of our friends for Sunday brunch. I'm appreciative of those omelets and the originality that goes into putting 'em together. They're delicious.

So while simplicity is a delicious state of being, so is complexity, especially when the results satisfy the soul.

CULTURED ÇILBIR EGGS (TURKISH EGGS)

MAKES **1 SERVING**
5.8 MG PER SERVING

2 garlic cloves, smashed and peeled

½ teaspoon kosher salt

1 cup Greek yogurt, at room temperature

1 tablespoon chopped fresh parsley

2 large eggs

1 tablespoon distilled white vinegar

2 tablespoons butter

1 tablespoon olive oil

1 tablespoon Harissa Paste (recipe follows)

For garnish: chopped fresh cilantro and red pepper flakes

Toasted bread, for serving

1 In a bowl, muddle the garlic cloves and salt together until it forms a paste. Add the Greek yogurt and parsley. Set aside.

2 Set a fine-mesh sieve over a bowl. Crack one egg into it. Swirl it gently so that the watery part of the egg white drips into the bowl below. (This step is to prevent the whites from dispersing in the poaching water to give you better looking eggs.) Repeat this for the second egg and gently transfer the eggs to two separate ramekins. Set aside.

3 Line a plate with paper towels and have near the stove. Bring a medium saucepan of water to a simmer over medium-high heat. When the water begins to simmer, add the vinegar. Gently slide the eggs into the poaching water one by one. Reduce the heat and cook until the whites are set, 2 to 3 minutes.

4 With a slotted spoon, remove the poached eggs from the water and place them on the paper towels. Set aside.

5 In a small saucepan, melt the butter over medium heat. Stir in the olive oil and harissa paste and cook for 5 to 10 seconds. Remove from the heat.

6 To serve, top the bowl of yogurt mixture with the poached eggs. Generously drizzle the eggs and yogurt mixture with the spiced butter. Garnish with chopped cilantro and pepper flakes. Serve with toasted bread.

HARISSA PASTE

MAKES **1½ CUPS** (24 TABLESPOONS)
5.8 MG PER SERVING (I TABLESPOON)

4 dried guajillo chiles

2 dried ancho chiles

1 dried pasilla chile

2 teaspoons ground árbol chiles

2 tablespoons tomato paste

6 ounces jarred red bell peppers, roasted

4 large garlic cloves, peeled but whole

1 teaspoon caraway seeds, toasted and ground

2 teaspoons ground coriander

2 teaspoons ground cumin

1 teaspoon smoked paprika

½ teaspoon cayenne pepper

2 tablespoons fresh lemon juice

Kosher salt

2 tablespoons good-quality extra-virgin olive oil

1 tablespoon Cannabis Avocado Oil (page 10)

1 In a bowl, combine the dried chiles with hot water to cover and allow them to soak for 30 minutes or until the chiles are supple and rehydrated.

2 Stem and seed the chiles and add to a food processor. Add the tomato paste, roasted red peppers, garlic, ground caraway seeds, coriander, cumin, smoked paprika, cayenne, lemon juice, and a large pinch of kosher salt and blend. With the machine running, drizzle in the olive oil and the cannabis oil. Scrape down the sides intermittently as needed.

3 Adjust the seasoning if necessary. Transfer the harissa paste to a screw-top jar and refrigerate. The flavor will deepen after a few days.

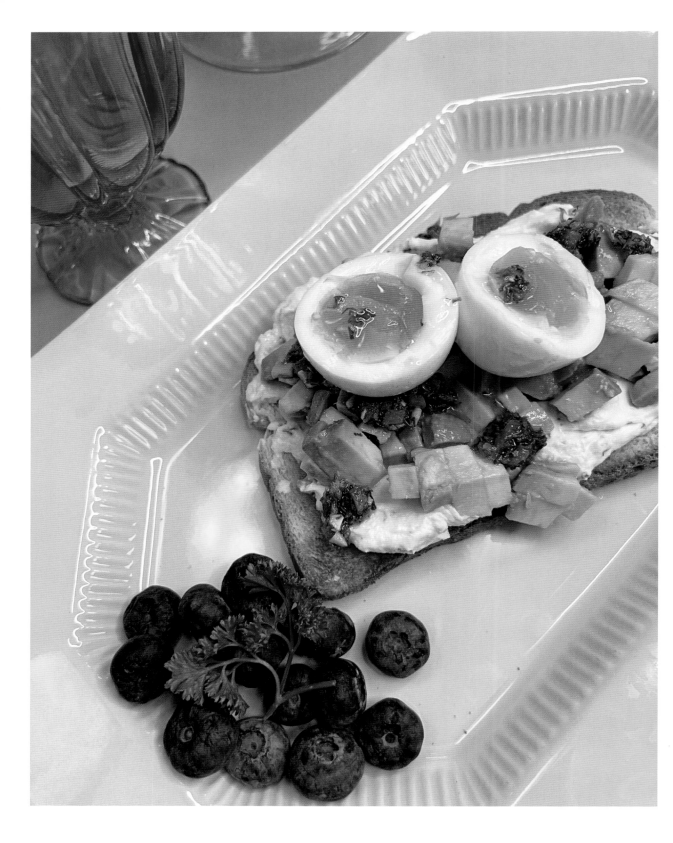

CREAMY EGG & AVOCADO TOASTS

MAKES **2 SERVINGS**
8.8 MG PER SERVING (2 TOASTS)

2 avocados, cubed

2 teaspoons fresh lime juice

Kosher salt

4 ounces mascarpone cheese

1 teaspoon garlic powder

1 tablespoon chopped fresh parsley, plus more for sprinkling

½ shallot, finely chopped

4 large eggs

4 thick slices country bread, toasted

4 tablespoons Chimichurri Special (page 87)

Freshly ground black pepper

1 tablespoon olive oil

1 In a small bowl, combine the avocado, lime juice, and a pinch of kosher salt. Set aside.

2 In another small bowl, mix the mascarpone cheese, garlic powder, 1 tablespoon chopped parsley, and shallot until well combined. Set aside.

3 Fill a medium bowl with ice and water and set near the stove. Bring a medium saucepan of water to a boil. Reduce the heat to a rapid simmer, gently add the eggs, and simmer for 6 minutes. Remove from the pan and place directly into the ice bath to halt the cooking. Drain and then peel.

4 Spread each slice of toast with one-quarter of the mascarpone mixture. Dividing evenly, add an even layer of the avocado.

5 Roughly chop the peeled eggs and add 1 to each of the 4 slices of toast. Top each toast with a tablespoon of chimichurri. Garnish with the remaining parsley, black pepper, a drizzle of olive oil, and salt to taste.

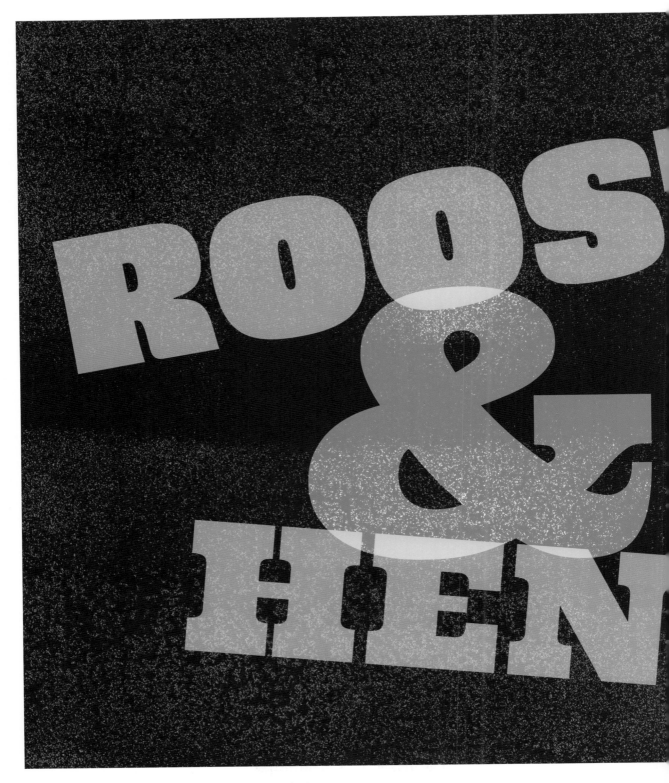

ERS

W

S

When Ray Price sang "Night Life," he turned it into a hit and suddenly put me on the map as a songwriter. We became forever friends, although that friendship was strained for a while. The cause was Ray's prize rooster.

It happened on my farm near the Kentucky/Tennessee border. I was raising pigs while Shirley, my second wife, was raising hens that she loved so much she gave each a name. Ray was going on tour and asked if I'd house his rooster. Sure thing. Turned out the rooster was aggressive and killed Shirley's favorite hen. Shirley raised such hell that I called Ray and told him to come by and pick up his animal. But Ray kept postponing the pickup. After the rooster killed a third hen, Shirley was beside herself. So I shot the damn rooster and we had him for supper.

Ray was furious. I explained that one good laying hen is worth five prize roosters. Didn't matter to Ray. He stopped talking to me . . . until I got him a prize bull at auction and dropped it off at his house in a trailer. A few days later, we had dinner and all was forgiven. Here's what we might have had.

BUTTER-BASTED CORNISH HENS WITH HERBED GRAVY

MAKES **4 SERVINGS**
30.2 MG PER SERVING

5 medium lemons

¼ cup fresh rosemary leaves, chopped, plus 10 (4-inch) sprigs

2 tablespoons fresh thyme leaves, chopped, plus 10 (4-inch) sprigs

1 tablespoon kosher salt, plus more to taste

1½ teaspoons freshly ground black pepper, plus more to taste

1 teaspoon sweet paprika

20 garlic cloves, smashed and peeled

8 tablespoons (4 ounces) butter, at room temperature

1 tablespoon Cannabis Ghee (page 9), at room temperature

2 Cornish hens (1½ to 2 pounds each), fresh or thawed frozen, giblets removed

1 tablespoon all-purpose flour

2 cups chicken broth

1 Squeeze 1 lemon to yield 2 tablespoons juice. Cut 1 lemon into 6 wedges and the remaining 3 lemons in half crosswise. Set aside.

2 In a food processor, combine the lemon juice, chopped rosemary, chopped thyme, salt, pepper, paprika, and 10 of the garlic cloves and process until the garlic is finely chopped.

3 In a bowl, combine the 8 tablespoons butter and cannabis ghee. Add the garlic/herb mixture and use a rubber spatula to fold until the ingredients are well combined.

4 Divide into 2 equal portions and carefully stuff the compound butter under the skin of the hens. Fill each cavity with 3 lemon wedges and 5 garlic cloves. Truss each hen with kitchen twine by tying together the legs.

5 Arrange the rosemary sprigs and thyme sprigs in an even layer in a large roasting pan. Place the hens on top of the herb sprigs and allow to rest at room temperature, uncovered, for 1 hour.

6 Meanwhile, preheat the oven to 425°F.

7 Cover the roasting pan with a lid or aluminum foil and roast for 25 minutes.

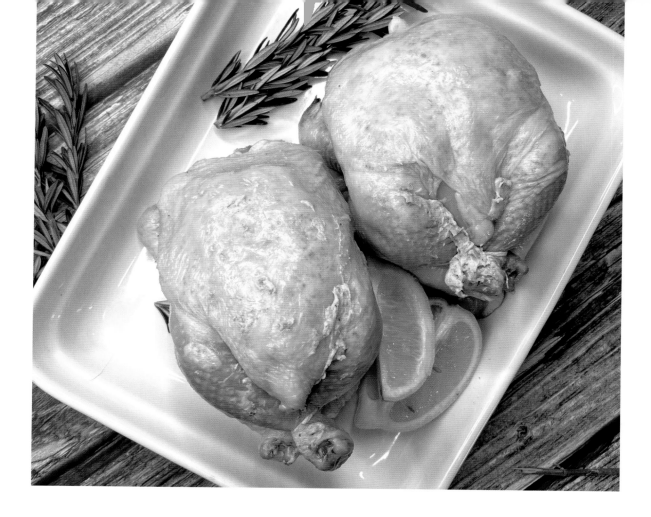

8 Uncover and continue roasting until the skin is golden brown and a thermometer inserted registers 165°F in the thickest part of the hen, 25 to 35 minutes, basting the hens with the drippings every 10 minutes.

9 Remove the hens from the roasting pan and set aside to rest.

10 Meanwhile, in a small bowl, stir together the flour and 1 cup of the chicken broth until smooth. Add the drippings to a saucepan and bring to a simmer over medium-low heat. Once at a simmer, whisk in the flour mixture and, as the gravy thickens, add the remaining 1 cup chicken broth. Simmer until it reaches the desired consistency. Season to taste with kosher salt and black pepper.

11 To serve, strain the gravy and serve with the Cornish hens that have been carefully halved.

COCOA COQ AU VIN

MAKES **4 SERVINGS**
20.8 MG PER SERVING

3 tablespoons olive oil, divided

4 ounces bacon, finely diced

8 bone-in, skin-on chicken thighs (about 4 pounds), trimmed of excess skin

Kosher salt and freshly ground black pepper

1 large yellow onion, roughly chopped

4 garlic cloves, chopped

¼ cup cognac

2½ cups pinot noir

2½ cups chicken broth, plus more as needed

1 tablespoon tomato paste

2 tablespoons black cocoa powder

2 cloves black garlic, left whole

2 teaspoons balsamic vinegar

1 tablespoon fresh thyme leaves

1 bay leaf

3 large carrots, peeled and cut into chunks on the bias

1½ teaspoons sugar

8 ounces cremini mushrooms, sliced

3 tablespoons unsalted butter, at room temperature

2 teaspoons Cannabis Ghee (page 9), room temperature

4 tablespoons all-purpose flour

1 Line a plate with paper towels and set near the stove. In a 5-quart Dutch oven or heavy-bottomed pot, heat 1 tablespoon of the oil over medium heat. Add the bacon and cook until the fat has rendered and the bacon is crispy. Using a slotted spoon, transfer the bacon to the paper towels, leaving the fat in the pan.

2 Season the chicken with 2 teaspoons salt and ½ teaspoon pepper. Increase the heat to medium-high and add half of the chicken, skin-side down, and cook until golden, about 5 minutes. Transfer the chicken to a plate. Repeat with the remaining chicken. Pour off all but 2 tablespoons of the fat from the pot.

3 Return the pot to the stove and reduce the heat to medium-low. Add the onion and cook until softened and just starting to brown. Add the regular garlic and stir until fragrant. Add the cognac, scraping up any browned bits from the bottom of the pan, and cook until the alcohol has evaporated. Add the wine, chicken broth, tomato paste, cocoa powder, black garlic, vinegar, thyme, bay leaf, and ½ teaspoon salt. Stir/whisk until the cocoa is incorporated. Bring to a boil, then reduce the heat to medium and cook, uncovered, for 10 minutes.

4 Return the chicken to the pot, along with any accumulated juices, and add the carrots and sugar. Bring to a simmer, cover, and cook over low heat until the chicken and carrots are cooked through, about 30 minutes.

5 Meanwhile, in a large skillet, heat the remaining 2 tablespoons oil over medium heat. Add the mushrooms and ¼ teaspoon salt and cook, stirring frequently, until the mushrooms are golden brown. Set aside.

6 In a small bowl, combine the softened butter, cannabis ghee, and flour to make a smooth paste. Set aside.

7 Transfer the cooked chicken and carrots to a plate.

8 Discard the bay leaf and thyme. With an immersion blender, blend the liquid ingredients and black garlic in the pot until smooth. (Alternatively, do this in a stand blender and then return the liquid to the pot.)

9 Increase the heat under the Dutch oven/pot to medium and stir in the cannabis butter/flour paste. Gently boil until the sauce is thickened. Add additional chicken broth for desired thickness/loosening of the sauce.

10 Remove the skin from the chicken and return the chicken thighs and any accumulated juices to the pot. Simmer, uncovered, for about 7 minutes.

11 Add the carrots, mushrooms, and rendered bacon.

THESE LITTLE PIGGIES

Somewhere in the lost years of the sixties, I fashioned myself a pig farmer. It was in the middle of a harsh winter when I bought seventeen weaner pigs for a quarter a pound and, genius that I am, wound up selling them six months later for seventeen cents a pound. I learned the hard way that pigs are smart. They found ways of escaping the pen and caused all sorts of grief. The picture of me chasing after those pigs is not a pretty sight.

Sometimes I have dreams where, instead of me chasing the pigs, the pigs are chasing me. Yet despite my disastrous experience with the animal, I harbor no grudge.

Pork is tasty. Whether you're chowing down on a pork sandwich at a roadside stand or cooking up a sweetly succulent pork dish, it's a flavorful meat with an attitude all its own.

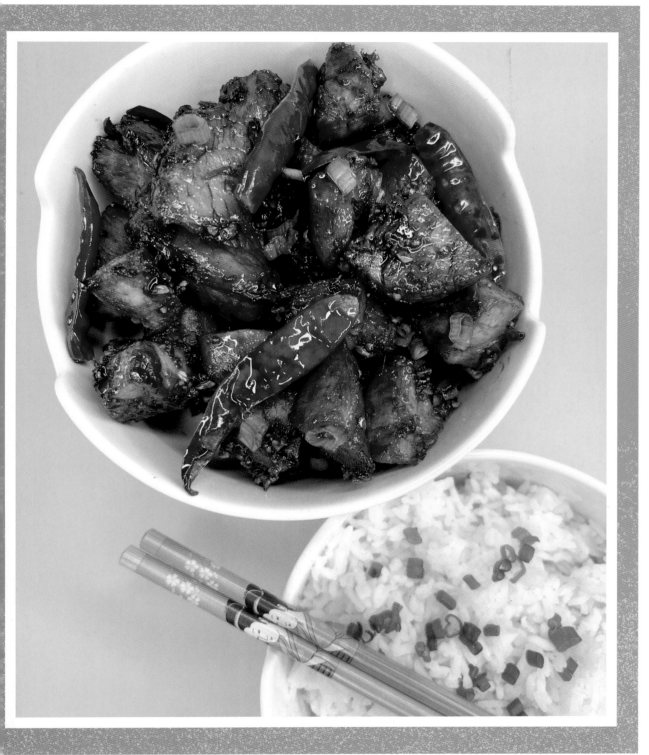

STICKY MISO
PORK BELLY

MAKES **6 SERVINGS**
23.5 MG PER SERVING

PORK BELLY

2½ pounds skinless pork belly, cut into cubes 1½ to 2½ inches long

4½ cups chicken stock

1 tablespoon minced fresh ginger

3 garlic cloves, minced

1 tablespoon rice vinegar

1 tablespoon sugar

GLAZE & GARNISH

1 tablespoon Cannabis Grapeseed Oil (page 11)

1 tablespoon minced fresh ginger

3 Thai chile peppers, finely chopped

3 tablespoons dark soy sauce

2 tablespoons honey

2 tablespoons light brown sugar

1 tablespoon lemongrass paste

2 teaspoons miso

Kosher salt and freshly ground black pepper

1 tablespoon vegetable oil

Sesame seeds, sliced scallions, and sliced chile peppers, for garnish

CHEF'S NOTE: Can be served over rice or as is.

1 PREPARE THE PORK BELLY: Place the pork belly in a Dutch oven and cover with the chicken stock. Add the ginger, garlic, rice vinegar, and sugar. Bring to a boil. Reduce to a simmer, cover, and cook until the pork cubes are tender, about 2 hours.

2 Drain the pork belly and pat dry. Cut the pork into bite-size chunks.

3 MAKE THE GLAZE: In a small bowl, mix together the cannabis oil, ginger, chiles, soy sauce, honey, brown sugar, lemongrass paste, miso, and salt and pepper to taste. Mix until well combined.

4 In a skillet, heat the vegetable oil over medium-high heat. Add the pork belly and season with salt and pepper to taste. Fry while turning regularly and until the pork belly is golden.

5 Pour the glaze over the pork and continue to cook for a couple of minutes, until the pork looks dark and sticky. Remove from the heat and garnish with scallions, sesame seeds, and more sliced chiles.

GRILLED PORK CHOPS WITH PINEAPPLE PICO DE GALLO

MAKES **4 SERVINGS**
11.75 MG PER SERVING

MARINATED PORK CHOPS

- ¼ cup olive oil
- ¼ cup reduced-sodium soy sauce
- 2 tablespoons pineapple juice
- 2 tablespoons brown sugar or honey
- 2 tablespoons Dijon mustard
- 3 garlic cloves, minced
- 1 teaspoon cayenne pepper
- 4 bone-in pork chops, at least 1 inch thick is best

PINEAPPLE PICO DE GALLO

- ½ cup diced pineapple
- ⅓ cup diced cherry tomatoes
- 3 tablespoons diced red onion
- 2 tablespoons chopped fresh cilantro
- 1 Thai chile pepper, finely minced
- 1 garlic clove, minced
- 1 teaspoon ground cumin
- 1 teaspoon garlic powder
- ½ lime
- Kosher salt
- 1 teaspoon Cannabis Avocado Oil (page 10)

1 MARINATE THE PORK CHOPS: In a bowl, combine the olive oil, soy sauce, pineapple juice, brown sugar, mustard, garlic, and cayenne. Whisk until thoroughly combined.

2 Transfer the pork chops to a large zip-seal bag and add the marinade. Seal the bag tightly and refrigerate overnight.

3 MEANWHILE, MAKE THE PINEAPPLE PICO DE GALLO: In a large bowl, combine the pineapple, tomatoes, onion, cilantro, chile pepper, minced garlic, cumin, and garlic powder and gently fold the ingredients together. Squeeze the juice from ½ lime over the ingredients. Add salt to taste and mix gently. Adjust the seasoning as needed. Fold in the cannabis oil until well combined. Cover and refrigerate for at least 1 hour before serving.

4 Once the chops have marinated, preheat an outdoor grill to 400°F (medium-high heat).

5 Remove the pork chops from the marinade (discard the marinade). Sear the pork chops on the grill for about 2 minutes per side.

6 Reduce the grill heat to medium and grill the pork chops until they reach an internal temperature of 145°F, 4 to 7 minutes per side.

7 Remove from the grill, cover with foil, and let rest for 5 minutes.

8 Serve with equal portions of the pico de gallo.

ON

ROAD

THE

AGAIN

SIMPLE & NOT SO SIMPLE SALMON

Annie makes me one of my favorite salmon dishes. It's a simple broiled salmon with a salt crust and finished with Bragg Liquid Aminos spray. Here are other ways to work up salmon—adventurous recipes from Andrea.

BROILED SALMON WITH WASABI AIOLI

MAKES **4 SERVINGS**
17.6 MG PER SERVING

½ cup mayonnaise

½ teaspoon garlic powder

1 teaspoon wasabi powder

½ teaspoon soy sauce

½ teaspoon Cannabis Grapeseed Oil (page 11)

4 skin-on salmon fillets (6 ounces each)

2 tablespoons olive oil

Maldon sea salt

Chopped fresh herbs, such as parsley, dill, or chives (optional), for serving

1 In a small bowl, stir together the mayo, garlic powder, wasabi powder, soy sauce, and cannabis oil. Refrigerate until ready to serve.

2 Position an oven rack so that it's about 6 inches from the broiler element at the top.

3 Line a large baking dish with parchment paper and arrange the fillets skin-side down so that they are not touching. Brush the fillets with the olive oil and season each with Maldon sea salt.

4 Broil the fillets until the salmon flakes easily when tested with a fork, it appears medium-rare in the center, and the internal temperature on an instant read thermometer inserted at the thickest part reads 135°F, 7 to 9 minutes (check early at the 6-minute mark to gauge progress). If you prefer your salmon well-done, leave it in for another minute or so, until the internal temperature reaches 140°F. DO NOT overcook. If at any point the top of the salmon starts to look too dark for your liking, loosely tent it with foil.

5 Allow the salmon to rest for 5 minutes. Top each fillet with 2 tablespoons wasabi aioli. If desired, garnish with fresh herbs.

JAMAICAN JERK SALMON

MAKES **6 SERVINGS**
23.5 MG PER SERVING

1 side of salmon
   (2½ pounds)
Kosher salt
1 cup Jerk Marinade
   (recipe follows)

1 Position a rack in the center of the oven and preheat the oven to 325°F.

2 Place the salmon in a large baking dish and pat dry with a paper towel to remove moisture. Season both sides with kosher salt and refrigerate uncovered for 15 minutes.

3 Remove the salmon from the fridge, add the jerk marinade to the salmon, massaging it in for full coverage. Refrigerate for another 15 minutes.

4 Bake the salmon until the thickest part flakes easily when tested with a fork, 30 to 35 minutes.

5 Let rest for 5 minutes before serving. Serve warm or at room temperature.

JERK MARINADE

MAKES **2 CUPS** (32 TABLESPOONS)
8.8 MG PER TABLESPOON

1 medium onion, quartered

5 scallions, halved crosswise

1 bunch thyme, leaves picked

12 to 15 garlic cloves, peeled but whole

2 Scotch bonnet or habañero peppers

1 small knob fresh ginger

10 allspice berries

2 teaspoons smoked paprika

1 teaspoon ground cinnamon

1 teaspoon freshly grated nutmeg

¼ teaspoon ground allspice

⅛ teaspoon ground cloves

3 tablespoons light brown sugar

2 tablespoons soy sauce

½ tablespoon browning liquid

Juice of 1 lemon

Juice of 1 orange

2 tablespoons Cannabis Grapeseed Oil (page 11)

In a food processor, combine all the ingredients and pulse until finely pureed. Store in a glass jar in the refrigerator. For added shelf life, freeze in ice cube trays and transfer to a freezer bag once frozen.

SALMON

>> 1981, in North Finland. A little town named Ivalo, twelve hours north of Helsinki, not far from the Russian border. Dead of winter.

I was up there doing the TV film *Coming Out of the Ice* starring John Savage. My role was Red Loon, a political prisoner stranded in Siberia.

The crew and actors stayed in remote little huts along the Ivalo River. Lake Salmon provided our nightly meal—salmon stew.

But then things changed when one afternoon

we were out on our cross-country skis, checking out the vast white wilderness, when we saw our chef hit a reindeer with his car. It was tough to say whether it was intentional or inadvertent. All I know is that, from then on out, the big switch was from salmon to reindeer chops.

Given the freezing climate, I was grateful for any food piping hot.

STEW

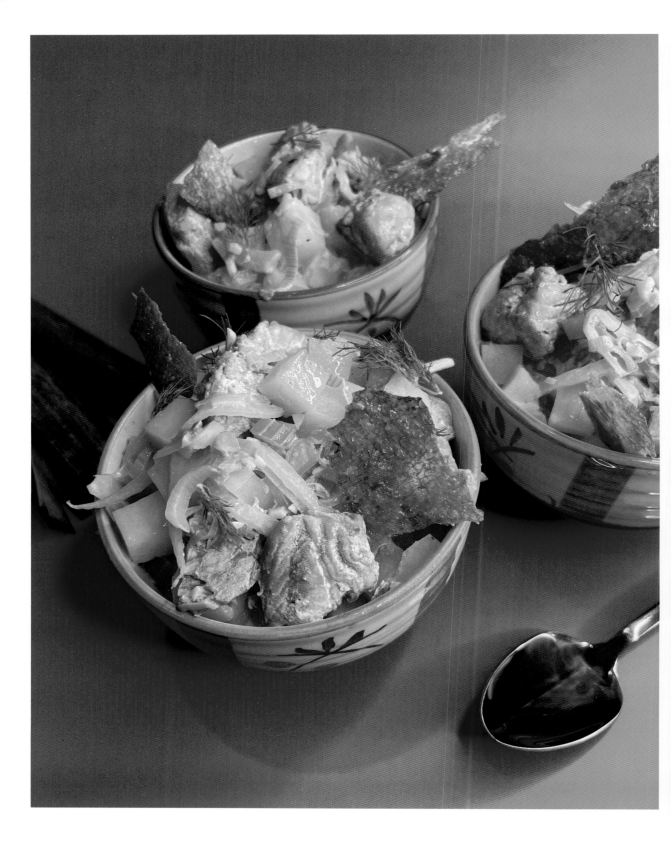

SALMON CHOWDER

MAKES **6 SERVINGS**
35.3 MG PER SERVING

2 leeks

2 tablespoons olive oil

1 tablespoon Cannabis Ghee (page 9)

1½ cups finely sliced fresh fennel

1 cup diced celery

4 garlic cloves, minced

1 teaspoon fennel seeds

2 teaspoons fresh thyme, minced

½ teaspoon smoked paprika

⅓ cup cooking sherry

3 cups fish stock

1 teaspoon kosher salt

1 bay leaf

¾ pound baby potatoes, medium diced

1 pound skinless salmon

Kosher salt

1 cup heavy whipping cream

Fennel fronds, for garnish

Lemon wedges, for squeezing

1 Slice the leeks into thin rounds and soak in cold water; drain and repeat process twice until the leeks are clean. Drain and set aside.

2 In a Dutch oven, heat the olive oil and cannabis ghee over medium heat. Add the leeks, fresh fennel, and celery and sauté until fragrant. Add the garlic, fennel seeds, and thyme and continue to sauté for an additional 3 minutes.

3 Stir in the smoked paprika and then the cooking sherry. Allow the alcohol to cook off for 2 minutes.

4 Add the fish stock, salt, and bay leaf and bring to a simmer over high heat. Add the potatoes and stir. Reduce the temperature to medium-low, cover, and cook until the potatoes are firm-tender. Take care not to overcook the potatoes.

5 Meanwhile, slice the salmon into 2-inch pieces, trimming any brown fat and removing bones, if necessary. Season lightly with kosher salt.

6 Once the potatoes are 2 minutes from done, add the heavy cream and salmon pieces. Cook for about 2 minutes, making sure the chowder is at a low simmer, but not boiling, allowing the salmon to gently poach while completing the cook on the potatoes.

7 Turn the heat off and allow the residual heat to finish cooking the fish. Using a fork, flake the fish apart, into bite-size pieces.

8 Adjust the seasonings as needed. Garnish with fennel fronds. Serve with lemon wedges.

GRILLED BBQ SOCKEYE SALMON

MAKES **8 SERVINGS**
17.6 MG PER SERVING

Pineapple BBQ Sauce
   (recipe follows)
2 tablespoons soy
   sauce
2 tablespoons honey
2 garlic cloves,
   minced
1 teaspoon fresh
   thyme, minced
10 lemons, cut into
   ¼-inch-thick slices
1 (2-pound) skin-on
   Alaskan sockeye
   salmon fillet

1 Prepare a charcoal or gas grill for direct cooking over medium-high heat.

2 Set half of the BBQ sauce aside for serving. In a bowl, combine the remaining BBQ sauce with the soy sauce, honey, garlic, and thyme. Set near the grill.

3 Oil the grill grates. Lay the lemon slices on the grill grate to create a bed for the salmon. Spread them out and overlap the slices.

4 Pat the salmon dry and place it on top of the lemon bed. Brush with half the BBQ sauce mixture and grill until the fish flakes easily when tested with a fork, 15 to 20 minutes, brushing with the remaining sauce halfway through.

5 Serve with the reserved BBQ sauce.

PINEAPPLE BBQ SAUCE

YIELDS **1 QUART** (4 CUPS)
SERVING SIZE **1 TABLESPOON**
MAKES **64 SERVINGS**
6.6 MG PER SERVING

1 tablespoon
    Cannabis Avocado
    Oil (page 10)
1 garlic clove,
    minced
½ medium sweet
    onion, minced
1 teaspoon kosher
    salt
2 cups tomato paste
8 ounces canned
    pineapple chunks
¾ cup pineapple juice
3 tablespoons
    molasses
3 tablespoons apple
    cider vinegar
2 tablespoons light
    brown sugar
2 tablespoons Dijon
    mustard
2 tablespoons
    Worcestershire
    sauce
2 tablespoons chili
    garlic paste

1 In a medium saucepan, heat the cannabis oil over medium heat. Add the garlic, onion, and salt and sauté until soft.

2 Add the tomato paste, pineapple chunks, pineapple juice, molasses, vinegar, brown sugar, mustard, Worcestershire sauce, and chili garlic paste. Simmer uncovered, stirring often, for about 15 minutes.

3 Remove from the heat and use an immersion blender to process until smooth.

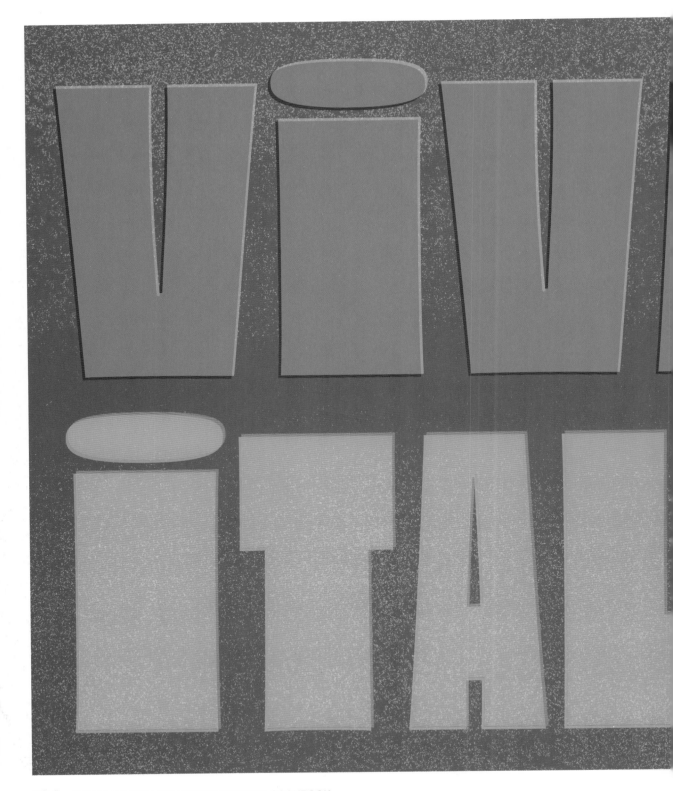

My wife, Annie, is a Sicilian cook who learned from her nonna. When we sit down to eat at our table, there is always an abundance of food.

Annie and I had some time off during a European tour and we got the boys together and we all rode on one bus through Europe. I woke early one morning when we were riding through Italy. I looked out the window and as far as the eye could see were fields of *girasole*. I went in to get Annie and we stood speechless for the longest time staring out at the sunflowers. That night on the bus we had one of her best cacio e pepes I can remember. It's a great dish when done just right.

PICI CACIO E PEPE

MAKES **4 SERVINGS**
17.6 MG PER SERVING

1 cup diced guanciale

2½ tablespoons olive oil

1½ teaspoons Cannabis Avocado Oil (page 10)

2 cups plus 2 tablespoons Italian tipo "00" flour

⅔ cup warm water

Kosher salt

2½ cups finely grated Pecorino-Romano cheese

1 teaspoon freshly ground black pepper

1 In a cast-iron skillet, render the diced guanciale over medium heat until the pieces are golden and crispy. Set aside at room temperature.

2 In a small bowl, stir together the olive oil and cannabis oil. Mound the flour on an impeccably clean work surface and make a well in the center. Add the olive oil mixture and warm water to the well and incorporate it into the flour using a fork until a rough dough forms.

3 Knead the dough for 10 minutes until it becomes smooth and elastic. Wrap in plastic wrap and allow it to rest at room temperature for 30 minutes.

4 Without adding additional flour to the work station, roll the dough out into a round ⅓ inch thick. Cut into ¼-inch-wide strips. Roll each strip out so that it resembles thick spaghetti. Again, do not dust your station with additional flour.

5 Transfer the rolled pici to a tray dusted with flour or semolina to prevent sticking.

6 Meanwhile, bring a pot of salted water to a boil, using less water than normal so that there will be a higher amount of pasta starch.

7 Add the fresh pasta to the boiling water and cook until 2 minutes shy of done. This step is important since the pasta will have additional cook time.

8 In a bowl, add a few ladles of starchy pasta water to the finely grated pecorino cheese in increments until it has the consistency of loose, creamy paste. Set aside.

9 In a large dry skillet, toast the black pepper over medium heat for 2 to 4 seconds. Add ½ cup pasta water and simmer while the pasta cooks.

10 Transfer the slightly undercooked pasta to the skillet with the pepper and stir briefly to release some of its starch.

11 Reduce the heat and add the pecorino mixture, stirring constantly until it transforms into a smooth and creamy cheese sauce. It may seem like it's going to split, but keep stirring until the texture changes. Once the mixture creams, turn off the heat and continue to stir for an additional minute to allow the sauce to thicken.

12 Serve garnished with the rendered guanciale.

LONG
&
WINDING
ROAD

In the beginning, the thought of bringing a chef on the road was an impossible dream. The early days were all about grabbing food at joints along the way. It wasn't until I was pretty well established—and that took forever—that I decided to hire a traveling cook.

The man called himself Beast. He came with his own bus he set up like a diner. I'd sit on a barstool at the counter while he worked the grill. I wasn't looking for haute cuisine. I was looking for bacon and eggs.

The Beast had perfected it—so much so that me and the boys had it for lunch, breakfast, and dinner.

That worked out well until, after a couple of years, I noticed I'd gained twenty-five pounds. Everyone else did too.

We were hooked on the Beast's bacon and eggs.

What to do?

Unfortunately, we had to let the Beast go.

But the story has a happy ending. The Beast went on to feed hundreds of other hungry musicians.

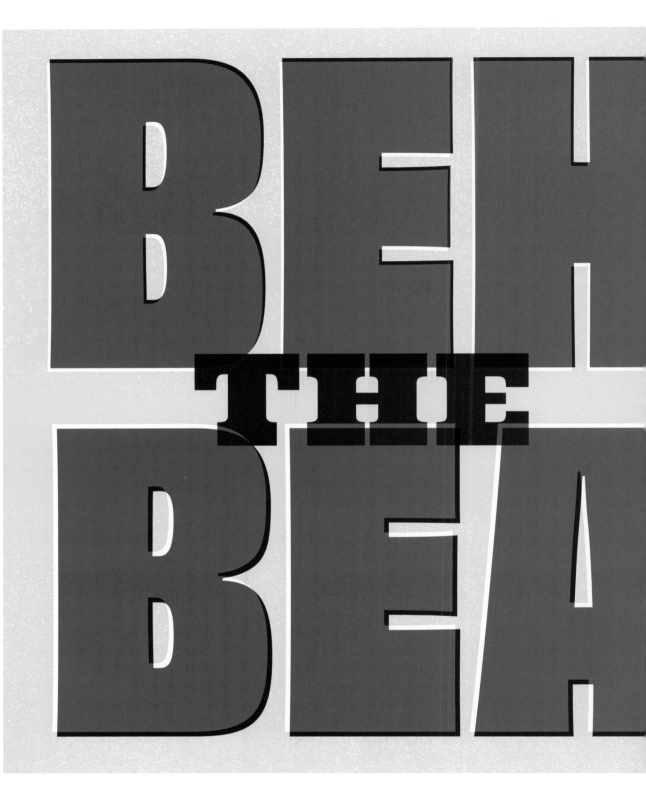

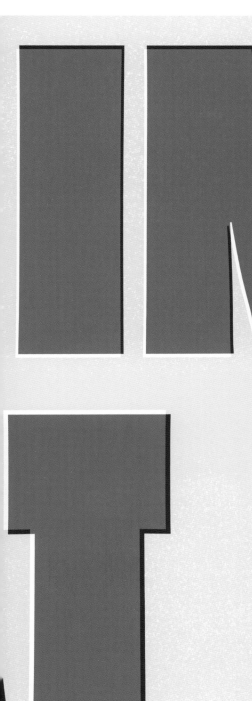

I sing behind the beat. Or ahead of the beat. Not sure which. But certainly not *on* the beat. I've always lived off the beaten track.

Same with food.

I remember seeing a fancy chart developed by a renowned nutritionist that determined what time of every day one should eat.

I looked it over and said to myself, "Hell, I eat when I'm hungry."

That schedule has always worked out for me.

I noticed, for example, when I first went to Spain, lots of folks don't start dinner till 10 at night. Or even later. That would give the nutritionist a nervous breakdown. But you know what? Eating-wise, the Spaniards have been doing okay for several centuries.

When I was hanging out in Madrid, all those late-night dinners were lots of fun, especially the night Annie and I were at the hotel and saw ten variations of egg dishes. Feeling adventurous, we tasted them all. Each was distinctive and delicious.

Andrea has her own take on a mouthwatering huevos rancheros.

CHILI HUEVOS RANCHEROS WITH ROASTED GARLIC & CHARRED ONION

MAKES **4 SERVINGS**
NO THC
(ADD **14.1 MG** PER SERVING FOR EVERY
3 TABLESPOONS CHILI SAUCE)

2 tablespoons rendered pork fat

2 tablespoons diced onion

1 tablespoon minced garlic

1 (15-ounce) can black beans, drained and rinsed

1 teaspoon ground cumin

Kosher salt

8 tortillas

Chili Sauce (recipe follows)

8 large eggs

Crumbled Cotija cheese, for serving

1 nopales paddle, grilled and diced

1 Roma tomato, diced

1 In a skillet, heat 1 tablespoon of the rendered pork fat over medium heat. Once hot, add the diced onion and cook until translucent. Add the garlic and cook until fragrant.

2 Add the black beans and cook until tender. Season with the cumin and kosher salt to taste. Use an immersion blender to mix the beans to a chunky mashed consistency. Set aside.

3 In another skillet, heat the remaining 1 tablespoon of pork fat over medium heat. Add four of the tortillas and lightly toast. Repeat with the remaining four tortillas. Cook the eggs over easy.

4 Spread 3 tablespoons of chili sauce on each of four plates. Place two toasted tortillas on each plate and top each tortilla with a spoonful of black beans and one of the eggs over easy. Finish with crumbled Cotija cheese, diced grilled nopales, and diced tomato.

CHILI SAUCE

MAKES **2 CUPS, 10 SERVINGS**
14.1 MG PER SERVING (3 TABLESPOONS)

1 small onion, charred

2 Roma tomatoes, charred

1 head garlic, roasted

3 dried ancho chiles

3 dried pasilla chiles

6 dried guajillo chiles

2 cups boiling water

2 teaspoons ground cumin

1 teaspoon Cannabis Grapeseed Oil (page 11)

⅓ cup chopped fresh cilantro

1 bouillon cube, chicken or vegetable

CHEF'S NOTE: This recipe requires only four servings of sauce. Store leftovers in a lidded jar in the refrigerator for up to 2 weeks.

1 Char the onion and tomatoes by setting over a high flame. You can use either a gas stovetop or an outdoor grill. Place the raw vegetables over the flame, rotating until evenly charred.

2 To roast the garlic, cut the top off the bulb to reveal the garlic cloves. Drizzle with oil and cover with foil. Roast in a preheated oven at 350°F for approximately 25 minutes or until the cloves are tender.

3 Place the dried chiles in a heatproof bowl and pour the boiling water over them to rehydrate. Set aside to soften.

4 Once the dried chiles are softened, drain and discard the water and add to a blender along with the charred tomato, charred onion, roasted garlic, cumin, cannabis oil, and cilantro. Blend until smooth. Transfer to a small saucepan.

5 Crumble the bouillon cube and add it to the saucepan. Cook over low heat until dissolved. Add water, if needed, to achieve the desired viscosity. Remove from the heat.

SPANISH NiGHTS

In the late nineties, Annie, our sons, and I were with the Kristofferson family in Almeria, Spain. Kris and I were filming *The Long Kill.* At night we'd sit by a crackling open fire as we ate fresh grilled meats and a delicious vegetable soup.

Deep memories: the sounds of haunting guitar pickin' and storytelling; the Andalusian mountains behind us; the Strait of Gibraltar in front of us; in the distance, the coast of North Africa.

The smell and feel of that salty dry air made time stand still.

KALE SOUP WITH SUN-DRIED TOMATOES

MAKES **2 SERVINGS**
17 MG PER SERVING

1 home-roasted red bell pepper

Canola or olive oil

4 ounces conchiglie pasta

2 tablespoons dairy butter or vegan butter

½ teaspoon Cannabis Ghee (page 9) or Vegan Cannabis Butter (page 9)

1 red onion, diced

3 tablespoons chopped sun-dried tomatoes, plus more (optional) for garnish

6 garlic cloves, minced

2 tablespoons tomato paste

4 cups vegetable stock

1 teaspoon dried sage

1 teaspoon dried basil

2 teaspoons chopped fresh parsley

½ cup roughly chopped kale, massaged

1 cup dairy heavy cream or vegan cream

Kosher salt and freshly ground black pepper

Rustic bread, toasted

1 Place the red pepper on a baking sheet and lightly oil. Roast in a 350°F oven for 15 minutes. Allow to cool. Chop and set aside.

2 Bring a pot of salted water to a boil. Add the pasta and cook according to the package directions. Drain and set aside.

3 In a heavy skillet, melt the butter and cannabis ghee over medium heat. Add the red onion, sun-dried tomatoes, and roasted pepper and cook until softened, 3 to 5 minutes.

4 Add the minced garlic and cook for an additional minute. Add the tomato paste and mix to evenly coat the skillet ingredients. Stir in the vegetable stock and mix thoroughly before adding the dried and fresh herbs.

5 Add the kale and cook for 2 to 3 minutes before adding the pasta to heat through. Remove from the heat and stir in the cream until well combined.

6 Garnish with black pepper and more sun-dried tomatoes, if desired. Serve with rustic toast.

GOAT
PART 1

I've always loved Jamaica. Jamaicans have big smiles, good hearts, delicious food, and great ganja.

One time I went to the island to record with Toots and the Maytals. I opened the door to my hotel room and there, across the pillow on the bed, was a bud the size of my arm. Welcome to Jamaica.

Next morning after breakfast, I returned to my room to find a fresh bud even bigger and prettier than the one from the day before. This went on for a week.

Meanwhile, me, Toots, and the Maytals made good music, had lots of laughs, and ate like kings. The chef kept a bottomless pot of goat stew simmering for us all week with heaping plates of sweet plantains and rice.

The memory is so strong and sweet that, as I write, I'm considering making a quick run to that enchanted island where the mixture of ganja and goat is irresistible.

CAJUN GOAT GUMBO

MAKES **10 SERVINGS**
14.1 MG PER SERVING

SPICE MIX

2 tablespoons sweet paprika

2 tablespoons garlic powder

1 teaspoon cayenne pepper

1 tablespoon dried thyme

1 tablespoon dried oregano

1 teaspoon celery seeds

1 teaspoon freshly ground black pepper

Kosher salt

GOAT GUMBO

3 quarts veal stock

1 cup peanut oil or bacon fat

1 tablespoon Cannabis Grapeseed Oil (page 11)

1¼ cups all-purpose flour

1 large green bell pepper, finely diced

2 medium onions, finely diced

4 celery stalks, finely diced

6 garlic cloves, minced

4 pounds boneless goat meat

1 pound smoked andouille sausage, cut into rounds

3 tablespoons grapeseed or other neutral oil

2 pounds fresh okra, split lengthwise

2 tablespoons filé powder

2 scallions per person

2 tablespoons chopped parsley per person

Cooked rice (optional), for serving

1 MAKE THE SPICE MIX: In a bowl, stir together the paprika, garlic powder, cayenne, thyme, oregano, celery seeds, black pepper, and salt to taste.

2 MAKE THE GOAT GUMBO: In a large pot, bring the veal stock to a gentle simmer over medium heat.

3 In a Dutch oven, heat the peanut oil and cannabis oil over medium heat. Whisk in the flour and stir frequently until it turns the color of chocolate, 15 to 25 minutes.

4 Add the bell pepper, onions, celery, and garlic and stir until well combined. Cook until the vegetables have softened.

5 Add the simmering stock one ladle at a time, whisking constantly until all of the stock has been thoroughly incorporated. Bring the mixture to a strong simmer over medium-high heat. Add the spice mix and stir until well combined.

6 Add the goat meat, reduce the heat to a simmer, cover, and cook until the meat is fork-tender, about 2 hours.

7 Transfer the meat to a bowl to cool. Then, using impeccably clean hands, shred the goat meat. You can also use forks to accomplish this process.

8 Return the meat to the gumbo sauce and add the andouille sausage. Cook for an additional 15 minutes.

9 Meanwhile, in a cast-iron skillet, heat the grapeseed oil over medium-high heat until sizzling hot. Working in batches, place the split okra in the skillet cut-side down. This will slightly soften the okra and sear it, preventing it from creating the signature texture familiar with okra.

10 Add the filé powder, the scallions, and parsley. Cook for an additional 3 minutes. Serve hot with rice or alone.

GOAT
PART 2

It was the seventies, and I was hanging out with Leon Russell, a certified genius if there ever was one. My bass player Bee Spears invited us to his place outside of Austin for dinner. Bee, who at the drop of a hat would spend $500 on pots and pans to whip up $5 worth of chili, told us he was cooking something extra special.

When we arrived, Bee was dragging the box spring of his king-size marital bed out to the backyard.

"What the hell are you doing?" Leon asked him.

"You'll see."

Well, an hour later he had turned that box spring into a fully functioning grill-over-a-pit. We didn't understand why the contraption had to be so big until Bee brought a goat. It was goat for dinner.

After dinner, I asked Leon what he thought.

"If you'd asked me before whether I thought grilled box spring goat would be any good, I would have said no. And I would have been wrong."

BRAISED GOAT AREPAS

MAKES **8 SERVINGS**
19.4 MG PER SERVING
(SUBTRACT 7.8 MG PER SERVING IF
NOT USING AVOCADO CREMA)

OVEN-BRAISED GOAT

3 pounds boneless goat meat

Kosher salt and freshly ground black pepper

2 tablespoons all-purpose flour

2 tablespoons extra-virgin olive oil

1 teaspoon Cannabis Grapeseed Oil (page 11)

2 medium carrots, chopped

2 medium shallots, chopped

4 scallions, roughly chopped

3 garlic cloves, chopped

2 tablespoons tomato paste

1 teaspoon chili powder

1 cup dry red wine

2 cups beef stock

2 tablespoons chopped cilantro

AREPAS

2 cups arepa flour (precooked cornmeal)

2 teaspoons kosher salt

2 tablespoons vegetable oil

1 teaspoon Cannabis Grapeseed Oil (page 11)

FOR SERVING

¼ cup crumbled Cotija cheese

Avocado Crema (recipe follows)

Lime wedges, for squeezing

1 MAKE THE OVEN-BRAISED GOAT: Preheat the oven to 325°F.

2 Pat the goat meat dry with paper towels and season liberally with salt and pepper. Sprinkle with the flour and coat evenly.

3 Heat a large Dutch oven over medium heat. Add the olive oil and cannabis oil, allowing it to get hot. Working in batches, sear the meat until golden brown on all sides. Transfer to a bowl and repeat the process with the remaining pieces of goat meat. Set the meat aside. Leave all of the oil in the pot.

4 Add the carrots, shallots, and scallions to the Dutch oven and sauté until softened. Return the goat meat to the pot and stir in the garlic, tomato paste, and chili powder. Cook for a minute and then add the red wine and beef stock.

5 Bring to a simmer, then cover and transfer to the oven. Braise until the meat is fork-tender, about 3 hours.

6 Remove the goat from the pot and allow it to cool. Shred the meat and set it aside.

7 Strain the braising liquid back into the pot and simmer until the sauce has reduced, discarding the carrots and scallions. Add the shredded meat to the pot and season with salt and pepper to taste. Stir in the chopped cilantro and set aside.

continues

BRAISED GOAT AREPAS

continued

CHEF NOTE: Pairs well with Avocado Crema.

8 MAKE THE AREPAS: In a medium bowl, stir together the arepa flour and salt. Make a well in the center of the arepa flour and add 2½ cups warm water. Stir together with a wooden spoon, stirring until there are no lumps. Allow the mixture to rest for 5 minutes. The dough should hold together easily.

9 Knead the dough in the bowl, then divide into 8 equal portions. Roll each portions on a clean work surface into a ball, then flatten into a round ½ inch thick.

10 In a small bowl, stir together the vegetable oil and cannabis oil. Heat a large nonstick skillet over medium heat, add 1 tablespoon of the oil mixture, and heat through. Add 4 of the arepas, cover, and cook until golden brown, about 6 minutes.

11 Uncover, flip, and continue to cook, uncovered, until golden brown, an additional 6 minutes. Transfer to a wire rack to cool. Repeat with the remaining arepa dough, adding additional oil if needed.

12 TO SERVE: Use a sharp knife to split the arepas and stuff with an equal portion of braised goat meat.

13 Sprinkle with crumbled Cotija cheese and serve with wedges of lime for squeezing and, optionally, avocado crema.

AVOCADO CREMA

YIELDS **1½ CUPS** (24 TABLESPOONS)
MAKES **12 SERVINGS**
7.8 MG PER SERVING (2 TABLESPOONS)

2 avocados, halved and pitted

Juice of 1½ limes

½ cup Mexican crema

2 teaspoons Cannabis Avocado Oil (page 10)

¼ cup chopped fresh cilantro (optional)

1 garlic clove, peeled but whole

1 teaspoon ground cumin

½ teaspoon smoked paprika

½ teaspoon kosher salt

¼ teaspoon garlic powder

Scoop the avocado into a blender or food processor. Add the lime juice, crema, cannabis oil, cilantro (if using), garlic, cumin, smoked paprika, salt, and garlic powder and blend until smooth, scraping the sides down as needed. Transfer to a jar or a squeeze bottle and refrigerate until ready to serve.

I NEVER WA

ID

Annie makes me a waffle almost every day.

   I like 'em with chicken-fried steak and gravy.

   I like 'em with ice cream.

   I like 'em with maple syrup.

   And I especially like the waffles I ate in Belgium.

   I was there for a gig and the club owner sent a whole batch of waffles to our bus for two straight days. Fluffy on the inside, crispy on the outside, they came with a heap of fresh berry preserves. Hands down, the world's best waffles.

   Here's a recipe that's world class.

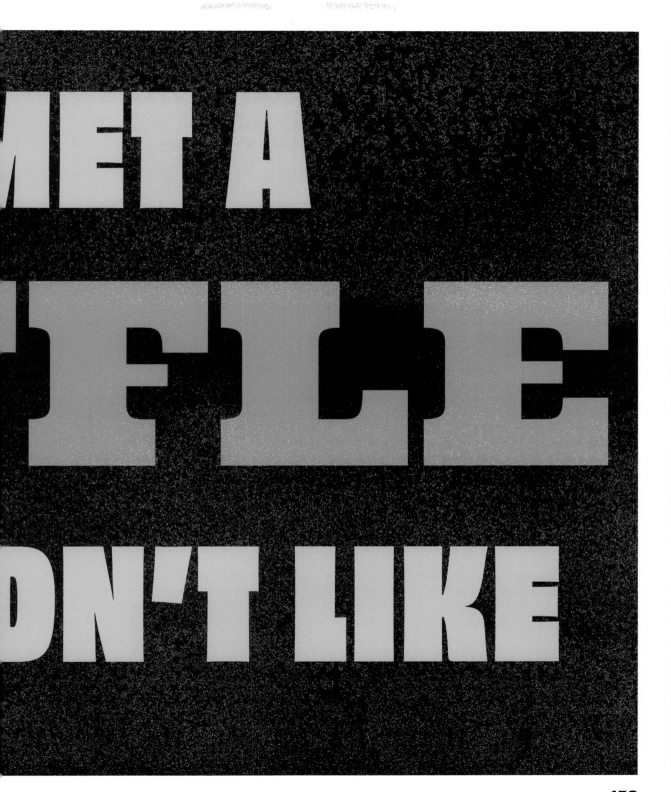

MET A

TFLE

ON'T LIKE

LEMON THYME LIÈGE WAFFLES

MAKES **10 WAFFLES**
21.1 MG PER SERVING (1 WAFFLE)

½ cup whole milk, at
room temperature

1 tablespoon instant
yeast

2 large eggs,
beaten, at room
temperature

2 tablespoons
Preserved Meyer
Lemon Paste

2 tablespoons honey

2 tablespoons fine
sugar

3 tablespoons fresh
thyme leaves

¾ teaspoon kosher
salt

3⅔ cups bread flour

15 tablespoons
(7½ ounces)
unsalted butter,
cubed, at room
temperature

1 tablespoon
Cannabis Ghee
(page 9), at room
temperature

1½ cups pearl sugar

Blueberry Compote
(recipe follows),
for serving

Whipped cream,
for serving

CHEF'S NOTE: You may also transfer
the waffles to a baking sheet and keep
warm in a 200°F oven for later. Waffles
should be served warm so the sugar
pearls don't crystallize. These waffles
pair well with blueberry compote.

PLEASE NOTE: THC mg increases
significantly to 44.5 mg per serving
if a serving of blueberry compote is
included. Recommended for the high-
tolerance consumer.

1 In a stand mixer fitted with the dough hook, combine the milk, ⅓ cup room-temperature water, the yeast, eggs, lemon paste, honey, sugar, thyme, and salt. Mix until well combined.

2 On low speed, add 2⅔ cups of the flour and mix until combined. On low speed, add the cubed butter and cannabis ghee, one cube at a time. Thoroughly mix in each added cube of butter and scrape down the bowl as needed. Once the butter has been incorporated, add the remaining 1 cup flour and knead on low speed until the dough is smooth and elastic.

3 Transfer the dough to a lightly oiled bowl and cover tightly. Set aside until the dough doubles in size, about 2 hours.

4 Punch the dough down, cover tightly again, and refrigerate overnight.

5 Preheat a Belgian waffle iron. (You can also use a regular waffle iron.)

6 Remove the dough from the fridge and knead in the pearl sugar. Divide the dough into 10 equal portions and roll each into a ball.

7 Place a ball of dough in the center of the waffle iron, close, and cook according to the manufacturer's instructions until golden all over.

8 Serve immediately, while still warm. Dividing evenly, top each waffle with warm blueberry compote and freshly whipped cream.

BLUEBERRY COMPOTE

YIELDS **4 CUPS**
SERVING SIZE ½ **CUP**
MAKES **8 SERVINGS**
23.4 MG PER SERVING

2 teaspoons
Cannabis Avocado
Oil (page 10)
or Cannabis
Grapeseed Oil
(page 11)

Grated zest of
1 lemon

4 cups blueberries

½ cup agave syrup

¼ cup water

2½ tablespoons fresh
lemon juice

½ vanilla bean, split
lengthwise, or
1 teaspoon vanilla
extract

1 In a saucepan, warm the cannabis oil over medium heat. Fold in the lemon zest and stir for 6 seconds.

2 Add 2 cups of the blueberries, the agave syrup, ¼ cup water, and the lemon juice. Scrape the vanilla seeds into the saucepan (if using extract, don't add yet). Simmer over medium heat for 10 minutes, stirring occasionally.

3 Add the remaining 2 cups blueberries and cook, stirring occasionally, about 6 minutes. Remove from the heat and stir in the vanilla extract (if using). The compote will thicken as it cools. Store in the refrigerator.

DORCY
DELIVERS

There's nothing I'd change about being on the road and no place I'd rather be. I'm never off the road too long without wanting to get back on it. I was on the road with Ray Price in the sixties when I met Ben Dorcy, the man they called "world's oldest roadie." He'd worked with everyone from John Wayne to Frank Sinatra. Fact is, he worked into his nineties. We liked him so well we called him Lovey.

He was our roadie when I did those Highwaymen tours with Waylon, Kristofferson, and Cash. Johnny was a prankster and liked to push Lovey to see how good he was really was.

Wish I could remember exactly where we were, but it was basically nowhere. Felt like the moon. The motel was empty except for us and our crews. The night was freezing cold. The four of us were shooting the shit in the lobby when Cash called up to Lovey's room and said, "Man, some crispy buttermilk fried chicken would sit real well about now."

It took him an hour, but Dorcy delivered. He showed up with two big buckets of crispy buttermilk fried chicken.

"Need anything else?" Lovey asked Johnny.

Johnny was speechless. All he could do was give Lovey a hug.

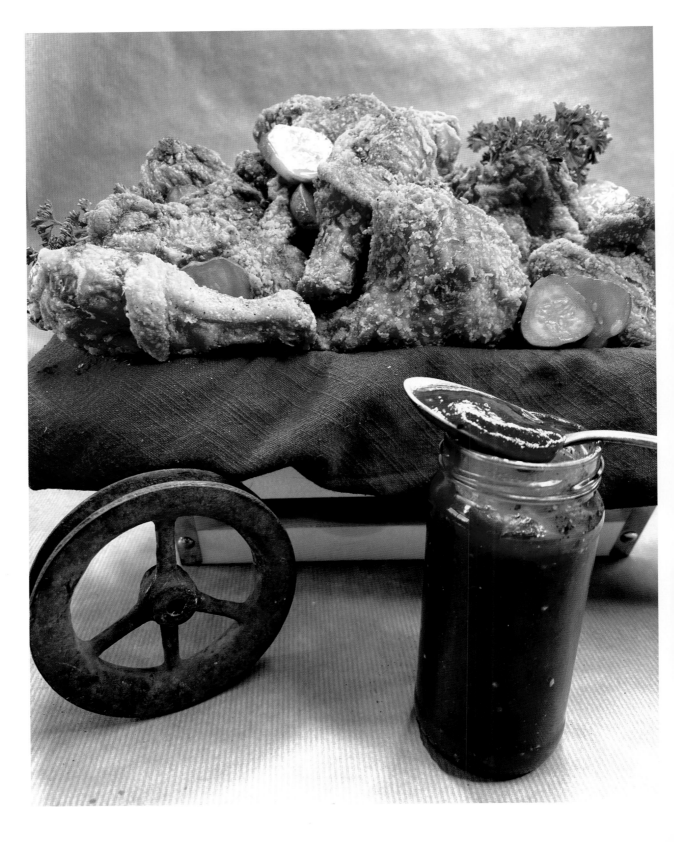

BUTTERMILK FRIED CHICKEN

MAKES **4 SERVINGS**
NO THC
(ADD **10.6 MG** PER SERVING FOR EVERY
I TABLESPOON MEMPHIS-STYLE BBQ SAUCE)

MARINATED CHICKEN

2 cups buttermilk

1 teaspoon kosher salt

1 teaspoon freshly ground black pepper

1 teaspoon garlic powder

1 teaspoon mustard powder

½ teaspoon smoked paprika

½ teaspoon dried thyme

8 pieces bone-in, skin-on chicken

DREDGE

2 cups all-purpose flour

1 tablespoon baking powder

1½ teaspoons salt

1½ teaspoons garlic powder

1½ teaspoons onion powder

1½ teaspoons smoked paprika

1½ teaspoons dried oregano

1½ teaspoons dried thyme

1 teaspoon adobo seasoning

1 teaspoon finely ground black pepper

ASSEMBLY

Grapeseed oil or other neutral oil, for frying

Memphis-Style BBQ Sauce (recipe follows), for serving

1 MARINATE THE CHICKEN: In a bowl, whisk together the buttermilk, salt, pepper, garlic powder, mustard powder, smoked paprika, and thyme until well combined. Place the chicken in a large zip-seal bag and pour in the buttermilk mixture. Seal tightly, removing any air in the bag, and refrigerate overnight.

2 MAKE THE DREDGE: In a shallow dish, whisk together the flour, baking powder, salt, garlic powder, onion powder, smoked paprika, oregano, thyme, adobo seasoning, and black pepper.

3 WHEN READY TO ASSEMBLE: Pour about two inches oil into a large cast-iron skillet and heat to about 340°F. Set a wire rack in a sheet pan and set near the stove.

4 Meanwhile, remove the marinated chicken from the fridge. Dredge each piece in the seasoned flour, gently pressing it onto the chicken for full coverage.

5 Once the oil reaches temperature, add the pieces in batches, careful not to overcrowd the skillet. Cook until golden brown and the internal temperature reads 165°F, 5 to 7 minutes. Transfer the cooked pieces to the wire rack to drain.

6 Serve with the Memphis-style BBQ sauce.

CHEF'S NOTE: BBQ sauce is intended for a dipping or basting sauce. To use as a basting condiment, add non-infused BBQ sauce to the recommended dose. Adding more per serving significantly increases THC levels.

MEMPHIS-STYLE BBQ SAUCE

MAKES 2½ CUPS (40 TABLESPOONS)
10.6 MG PER SERVING (1 TABLESPOON)

- 2 tablespoons Cannabis Ghee (page 9)
- 1 small onion, finely chopped
- 2 garlic cloves, minced
- 2 cups tomato sauce
- ½ cup apple cider vinegar
- ⅓ cup rice vinegar
- ⅓ cup molasses
- 3 tablespoons Worcestershire sauce
- 2 tablespoons dark brown sugar
- 2 teaspoons yellow mustard
- 1 teaspoon Louisiana-style hot sauce
- 1 teaspoon kosher salt
- 1 teaspoon freshly ground black pepper
- ¼ teaspoon cayenne pepper

1 In a medium saucepan, melt the ghee over medium heat. Add the onion and cook until softened. Add the garlic and cook until aromatic.

2 Add the tomato sauce, cider vinegar, rice vinegar, molasses, Worcestershire sauce, brown sugar, mustard, hot sauce, salt, black pepper, and cayenne and stir until fully combined. Bring to a boil. Reduce the heat to low and simmer, stirring occasionally, until slightly thickened.

3 Transfer the sauce to a blender and blend until smooth. Cool to room temperature and transfer to an airtight jar. Store in the refrigerator.

DINING

Thirty-six stories high. It was the early seventies. Producer Jerry Wexler was taking me to a restaurant atop a skyscraper in midtown Manhattan. A co-owner of Atlantic Records, Jerry helped me break out of the Nashville mold that never fit me right. He understood my music and I loved him. He gave me unchecked creative freedom and I gave him a song called "Shotgun Willie" where I talk about sitting around in my underwear and pulling out all my hair. Wex loved the song and wanted to celebrate.

"What do you feel like eating, Willie?" he asked.

"Something I've never eaten before."

"Great. I know the chef."

Wex knew everyone. He went off to the kitchen and came back smiling.

A few minutes later, the waiter served up an appetizer, crispy on the outside, soft on the inside. A little weird but tasty.

"Sweetbread?" I asked Jerry.

"Bull's balls. That bother you?"

I looked out the window. Manhattan was all aglow.

"Nope," I said before taking another big bite.

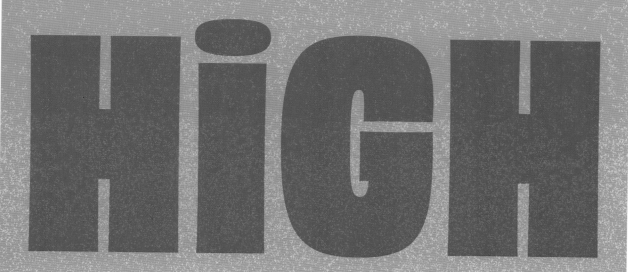

HiGH

ROCKY MOUNTAIN "SOYSTERS"

MAKES **24 "SOYSTERS"**
3.9 MG PER "SOYSTER"
(ADD **2.9 MG** PER SERVING WITH
SRIRACHA RANCH SAUCE)

3 cups mashed extra-firm tofu

1 cup shredded peeled Yukon Gold potato

¼ cup all-purpose flour, plus more as needed

2 teaspoons baking powder

¼ cup oat milk

2 teaspoons Cannabis Avocado Oil (page 10)

½ cup diced onion

1 teaspoon granulated garlic

1 tablespoon vegan beef base bouillon

1 teaspoon adobo seasoning

1 teaspoon soy sauce

1 teaspoon salt, or to taste

¼ teaspoon cracked black pepper

2 cups panko bread crumbs

2 tablespoons dried parsley

ASSEMBLY

1½ cups canola oil, for shallow-frying

Sriracha Ranch Sauce (page 164), for serving

Lemon wedges, for squeezing

CHEFS NOTE: Adding 1 serving of the Sriracha Ranch Sauce increases the dose to 6.8 mg per serving.

1 Wrap the tofu in an impeccably clean kitchen towel. Place on a solid surface and weight down with a heavy pot, pan, or books. Allow it to stand for 20 to 30 minutes. (If you have a tofu press, use that instead.)

2 Transfer the tofu to a bowl and mash with a fork or hands.

3 Squeeze any excess liquid from the shredded potatoes and add them to the mashed tofu.

4 In a separate bowl, mix together the flour, baking powder, oat milk, and cannabis oil until smooth. Pour the batter into the tofu mix. Add the diced onion, garlic, bouillon, adobo, soy sauce, salt, pepper, and 1 cup of the panko. Mix until thoroughly combined.

5 In a third bowl, mix together the remaining 1 cup panko and the dried parsley. Set the coating mixture aside.

6 Divide the tofu mixture into 24 equal portions and form into balls, then flatten into small discs. If the mixture is too loose, add additional flour 1 tablespoon at a time until the mixture is firmer and holds.

7 Dredge the cakes in the panko coating mixture.

8 Pour the canola oil into a cast-iron skillet and bring to 335°F over medium-high heat. Working in batches without overcrowding the skillet, cook the cakes until golden brown, 5 to 6 minutes. Drain on paper towels to absorb excess oil.

9 Serve with sriracha ranch sauce and lemon wedges for squeezing.

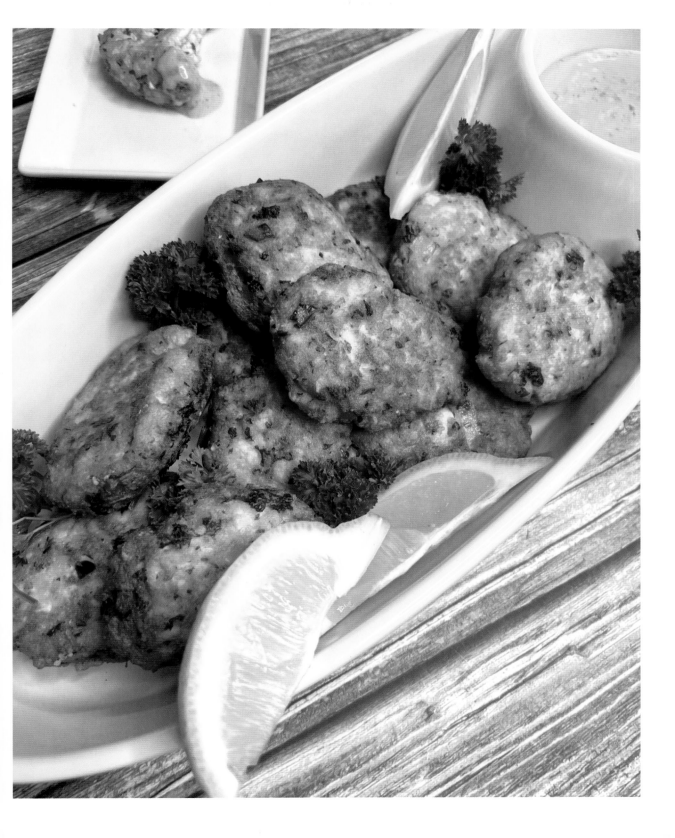

SRIRACHA RANCH SAUCE

YIELDS **1 CUP**
MAKES **8 SERVINGS**
2.9 MG PER SERVING (2 TABLESPOONS)

½ cup Cannabis-Infused Mayonnaise (recipe follows)

¼ cup whole milk (can be substituted with low fat or 2% or nondairy milk of choice)

2 tablespoons sriracha

1 tablespoon fresh lemon juice

1 tablespoon minced fresh flat-leaf parsley

1 tablespoon minced fresh chives

1 teaspoon minced fresh dill

1 teaspoon onion powder

1 teaspoon kosher salt

In a bowl, combine all the ingredients and mix thoroughly. Refrigerate for at least 1 hour before using.

CANNABIS-INFUSED MAVONNAISE

MAKES **1½ CUPS** (24 TABLESPOONS)
5.8 MG PER SERVING (2 TABLESPOONS)

1 large egg, at room temperature

1½ teaspoons fresh lemon juice

1 teaspoon white wine vinegar

¼ teaspoon Dijon mustard

¼ teaspoon sea salt

¾ cup plus 3½ tablespoons grapeseed oil

1½ teaspoons Cannabis Grapeseed Oil (page 11)

CHEF'S NOTE: You can also do this in a small food processor by slowly dripping the oil into the other ingredients as the machine is running. Start by dripping oil in a few tablespoons at a time until the mixture begins to emulsify, then slowly drizzle in the remaining oil.

1 In a wide-mouth jar or cup, combine the egg, lemon juice, vinegar, mustard, and salt. Pour in the oils and allow them to settle.

2 Place an immersion blender in the jar and press it firmly to the bottom, covering the egg yolk. Power on and keep it pressed against the bottom of the jar for at least 10 to 15 seconds.

3 Once the mixture begins to emulsify and thicken, slowly move the immersion blender up and down until the ingredients are thoroughly combined.

4 Transfer the mayonnaise to an airtight container and refrigerate.

1973: OUR FIRST FOURTH OF JULY PICNIC.

A 7,000-acre ranch at Dripping Springs, Texas.

Naysayers had their doubts.

No one would show up.

Well, tens of thousands of good folks *did* show up.

The rednecks and hippies would clash.

Well, they didn't. They got high and happy together.

No big stars would bother to come and perform.

Well, how about Loretta Lynn, Ernest Tubb, Kris Kristofferson, Rita Coolidge, and Asleep at the Wheel? They all showed up and sang.

The picnic became the template for decades of more 4th of July picnics to come. In fact, it became a major American musical tradition.

My favorite memory from that day was letting loose with Waylon, Leon Russell, and Doug Kershaw as we sang "Jambalaya."

Now that's a dish everyone loves.

JAMBALAYA

MAKES **8 SERVINGS**
17.6 MG PER SERVING

1 tablespoon Cannabis Grapeseed Oil (page 11)

10 ounces andouille sausage, sliced into rounds

1 pound boneless, skinless chicken thighs, cut into 1-inch pieces

1½ tablespoons Cajun seasoning

2 tablespoons vegetable oil

1 onion, diced

1 small green bell pepper, diced

1 small red bell pepper, diced

2 celery stalks, chopped

5 garlic cloves, minced

1 tablespoon crab paste

1½ tablespoons ground dried crayfish

1 (14.5-ounce) can San Marzano tomatoes

1 teaspoon kosher salt

½ teaspoon freshly ground black pepper

1 teaspoon dried thyme

1 teaspoon dried oregano

½ teaspoon red pepper flakes

2 teaspoons Worcestershire sauce

1 cup thinly sliced okra, or 1 teaspoon filé powder

1½ cups uncooked rice

3 cups chicken broth

1 pound Argentinian shrimp, peeled and deveined

1 pound crawfish tails

1½ cups cooked black-eyed peas

Sliced scallions, for garnish

1 In a large Dutch oven, heat the cannabis oil over medium heat. Season the sausage and chicken pieces with half of the Cajun seasoning.

2 Add the sausage to the hot oil and brown. Transfer to a bowl and set aside. Add the vegetable oil to the pot, add the chicken, and cook until lightly browned. Transfer to the bowl with the sausage and set aside.

3 Add the onion, both bell peppers, and celery and cook until the onion is soft and translucent. Add the garlic and cook until fragrant, about 30 seconds.

4 Stir in the crab paste and ground crayfish and sauté. Using your hands, break up the San Marzano tomatoes. Add salt, black pepper, thyme, oregano, pepper flakes, Worcestershire sauce, and the remaining Cajun seasoning.

5 Add the okra slices (or filé powder) and return the chicken and sausage to the pan. Be sure to incorporate the oils that the sausage and chicken were cooked in. Cook for 5 minutes, stirring occasionally.

6 Add the rice and chicken broth and bring to a boil. Reduce the heat to medium-low, cover, and simmer, stirring occasionally, until the liquid is absorbed and the rice is cooked, 20 to 25 minutes.

7 Place the shrimp and crawfish tails on top of the jambalaya mixture, stir through gently, and cover the pot. Simmer, stirring occasionally, until the shrimp and crawfish tails are cooked through. Add cooked black-eyed peas and allow to warm through.

8 Adjust the seasoning to taste and remove from the heat.

9 Garnish with sliced scallions. Serve hot.

FOOD &

& FUN

GROWING UP WITH FOREIGN FRIENDS

Growing up, me and sister Bobbie had friends from all walks of life—Mexican friends, Czechoslovakian friends, church friends, school friends, and even heathen friends.

We didn't think much about race unless it sat up right in our face and demanded attention. Like when Bobbie wanted to invite our rainbow of friends to see her play in church and was told no. That didn't make sense.

There were also some negative feelings about us Nelson kids playing places where folks drank beer and danced the polka. But, without saying it out loud, we knew in our hearts that all music is God's music, so we just followed the Lord's melody wherever it led.

If we hadn't played in those Czech barrooms, I'd never have my first go of goulash—and that'd be a damn shame.

GOULASH & DUMPLINGS

MAKES **8 SERVINGS**
35.2 MG PER SERVING

GOULASH

2 pounds beef chuck, cut into 1-inch pieces

Kosher salt and freshly ground black pepper

¼ cup grapeseed or avocado oil

2 tablespoons browning sauce

1 large onion, thinly sliced

4 carrots, diced

4 garlic cloves, minced

2 tablespoons sweet paprika

1 tablespoon tomato paste

1 teaspoon caraway seeds

2 tablespoons Cannabis Coconut Oil (page 10)

4 cups beef broth

1 (28-ounce) can whole peeled San Marzano tomatoes

1 teaspoon Worcestershire sauce

2 bay leaves

DUMPLINGS

½ cup all-purpose flour

¼ teaspoon freshly grated nutmeg

Kosher salt and freshly ground black pepper

½ cup whole milk

2 large eggs

12 ounces bread, cut into ½-inch cubes

6 ounces Gruyère cheese, shredded

3 scallions, finely chopped

ASSEMBLY

3 tablespoons olive oil

2 tablespoons minced garlic

2 fresh scallions, chopped

Freshly ground black pepper

1 Preheat the oven to 250°F.

2 **MAKE THE GOULASH:** Season the beef generously with salt and pepper. Heat a Dutch oven over medium-high heat and coat with the grapeseed oil. Working in batches, sear the beef until deep brown. Transfer to a bowl and toss with the browning sauce. Set aside.

3 Add the onion to the Dutch oven and cook, scraping any meat bits from the bottom of the pan. Add the carrots, garlic, and a pinch of salt and sauté until the onion is translucent. Add the paprika, tomato paste, and caraway seeds and stir until thoroughly combined. Cook for 2 minutes. Return the beef to the pan and add the cannabis oil, broth, tomatoes, Worcestershire sauce, and bay leaves and stir until combined.

4 Bring to a boil. Reduce to a simmer, cover, and transfer to the oven. Bake until the beef is tender and can be broken apart with a spoon but still maintains its shape, about 2 hours.

5 **MEANWHILE, MAKE THE DUMPLINGS:** In a small bowl, whisk together the flour, nutmeg, ¾ teaspoon salt, and a few grinds of black pepper.

6 In a large bowl, whisk together the milk and eggs. Add the bread cubes, Gruyère, and scallions and stir until thoroughly combined. Add the flour mixture and allow it to stand for 15 minutes.

CHEF'S NOTE: Using your hands, roughly crush the whole peeled tomatoes before adding.

7 Bring a large pot of salted water to a boil. Using a $\frac{1}{3}$-cup scooper, form firmly packed balls of the dumpling mixture and gently add them to the pot. Boil until cooked through, 15 to 20 minutes.

8 TO ASSEMBLE: In a large bowl, mix the olive oil, minced garlic, and scallions. Using a slotted spoon, add the cooked dumplings and coat generously with the mixture.

9 To serve, spoon the goulash into bowls and add a dumpling or two to each. Finish with black pepper to taste.

THE DELIGH

>> Annie makes beans and cornbread or a pot of chicken and dumplings to bring me back home. I consider dumplings comfort food. Soul food.

DUMI

IT

I imagine just about every culture has its version of dumplings. If you're dumpling-minded, here's a fresh twist on a dumpling dish you might find to your liking.

OF

PLINGS

COLLARD GREEN POTSTICKERS WITH PEANUT AGRODOLCE & CRISPY LACE

MAKES **3 SERVINGS**
15.6 MG PER SERVING (5 DUMPLINGS)

POTSTICKER FILLING

1½ cups thin strips collard greens (stems and midribs removed)

2 tablespoons olive oil

1 teaspoon Cannabis Avocado Oil (page 10)

¼ cup finely diced pancetta

2 tablespoons minced garlic

1 tablespoon minced fresh ginger

1 teaspoon smoked paprika

1 teaspoon red pepper flakes

2 tablespoons soy sauce

1½ teaspoons molasses

1 scallion, finely chopped, plus more for garnish

PEANUT AGRODOLCE

1 cup roasted peanuts

5 garlic cloves, roasted

Grated zest of 1 lime

4 tablespoons fresh lime juice

4 tablespoons honey

2 tablespoons balsamic vinegar

2 tablespoons sweet Calabrian chili powder

1 tablespoon Calabrian hot chili oil

POTSTICKERS & LACE SLURRY

15 wonton wrappers

⅓ cup water

2¼ teaspoons all-purpose flour

Pinch of kosher salt

2 tablespoons neutral oil

1 MAKE THE POTSTICKER FILLING: Set up a large bowl of ice and water and have near the stove. Bring a medium pot of water to a boil. Add the julienned collard greens and blanch for about 1 minute or until they turn a vibrant green. Using a set of tongs, transfer the greens to the ice bath to stop the cooking process. Drain and set aside.

2 In a skillet, heat 1 tablespoon of the olive oil plus the cannabis oil over medium heat. Once hot, add the diced pancetta and render until slightly crispy.

3 Add the minced garlic and ginger and cook until fragrant. Add the drained collard greens and sauté for 3 to 5 minutes. The greens will retain a lot of their texture.

4 Add the smoked paprika, pepper flakes, soy sauce, and molasses and sauté for 1 minute before adding the scallion. Remove from the heat and allow the mixture to cool.

5 MEANWHILE, MAKE THE PEANUT AGRODOLCE: Combine the whole roasted peanuts, garlic, lime zest, lime juice, honey, vinegar, chili powder, and chili oil in a blender and mix until smooth. Transfer to a small bowl and set aside.

CHEF'S NOTE: If you want to increase the dosage of this dish, substitute 1 teaspoon of the oil used in the lace slurry with cannabis oil.

6 COOK THE POTSTICKERS: Next, add 2 to 3 teaspoons of the cooled filling to each wonton wrapper and brush the edges of the wrapper with a wet finger. Fold to seal using a push and pinch technique to achieve small pleats in the stuffed wonton. Cover the 15 finished wantons with a damp napkin.

7 In a bowl, whisk ⅓ cup water, the flour, salt, and oil until smooth. Set the lace slurry aside.

8 In a large skillet, heat the oil over medium heat. Once heated, line the skillet with the 15 dumplings. Cook until the bottom of the wontons are golden and crispy, 3 to 5 minutes.

9 Whisk the lace slurry again and carefully pour it into the skillet from the side of the pan. Use caution as there will be some splatter. Make sure to distribute the slurry evenly, ensuring that all the spaces between the dumplings are covered with the mixture. Reduce the heat to medium, cover, and cook the dumplings for 5 to 6 minutes.

10 Uncover. If parts of the lace are still pale, move the pan so that the heat can focus on those areas until the water is fully evaporated. Once all of the dumpling lace is golden, turn off the heat.

11 Carefully place a large plate over the dumplings and hold in place while using your free hand to secure the handle. Carefully flip the laced dumplings onto the serving plate.

12 Garnish the lace with the peanut agrodolce and chopped scallions and serve immediately.

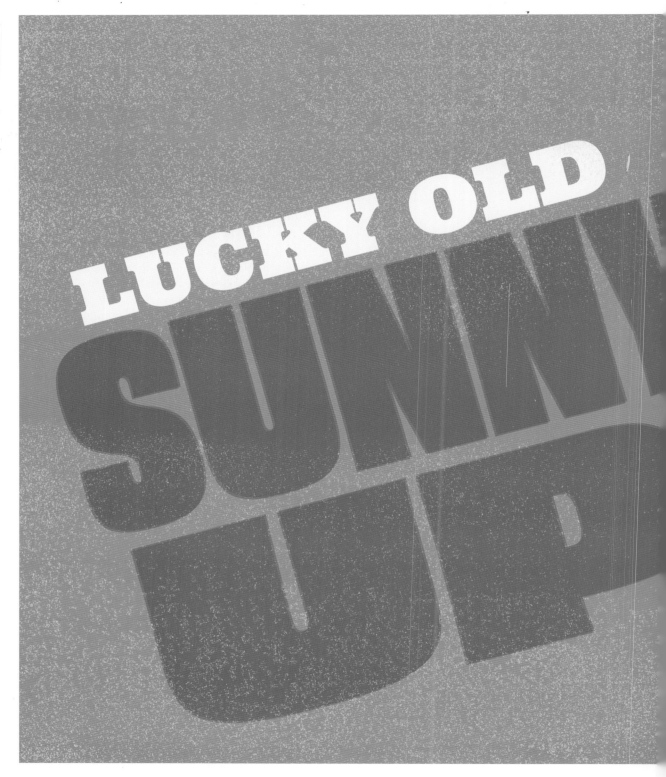

LUCKY OLD SUNNY UP

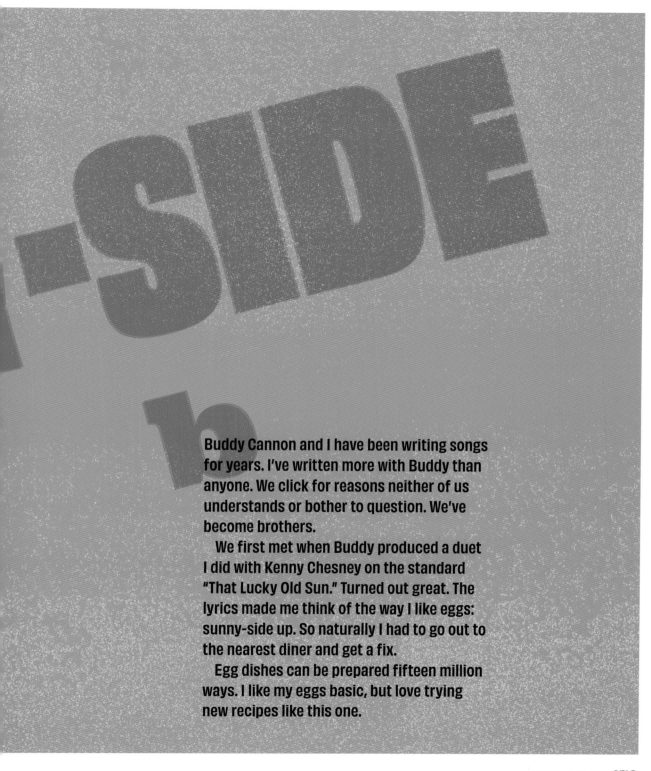

SIDE b

Buddy Cannon and I have been writing songs for years. I've written more with Buddy than anyone. We click for reasons neither of us understands or bother to question. We've become brothers.

We first met when Buddy produced a duet I did with Kenny Chesney on the standard "That Lucky Old Sun." Turned out great. The lyrics made me think of the way I like eggs: sunny-side up. So naturally I had to go out to the nearest diner and get a fix.

Egg dishes can be prepared fifteen million ways. I like my eggs basic, but love trying new recipes like this one.

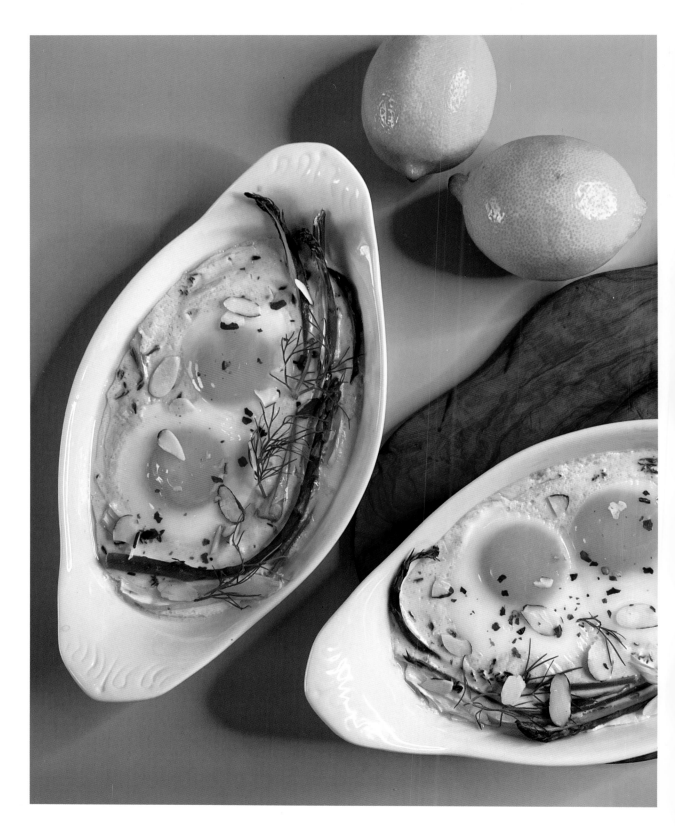

SHIRRED EGGS WITH ASPARAGUS & FENNEL

MAKES **2 SERVINGS**
17.6 MG PER SERVING

¼ pound asparagus, trimmed and thinly shaved

¼ pound fennel, thinly shaved

½ teaspoon Cannabis Ghee (page 9)

¾ cup heavy cream

1½ teaspoons Dijon mustard

1 teaspoon kosher salt

¼ teaspoon freshly ground black pepper

1 tablespoon fresh thyme, chopped, plus more for serving

4 large eggs

Pinch of red pepper flakes

1 tablespoon sliced almonds

1 teaspoon grated lemon zest

Maldon flaky sea salt

Rustic bread, toasted, for serving

1 Preheat the oven to 375°F.

2 Layer the shaved asparagus and fennel in two 16-ounce oval ramekins. Add ¼ teaspoon cannabis ghee to each.

3 In a small bowl, whisk together the heavy cream, mustard, salt, pepper, and thyme.

4 Pour half of the cream mixture over the shaved asparagus and fennel.

5 Make 2 small wells in each dish and carefully pour an egg into each. Drizzle the remaining cream over the egg whites, being cautious not to cover the yolks.

6 Transfer to the oven and bake until the egg whites are set and the yolks are cooked to specificity, 12 to 15 minutes.

7 Garnish with fresh thyme, pepper flakes, sliced almonds, lemon zest, and a sprinkle of Maldon salt. Serve with toasted rustic bread.

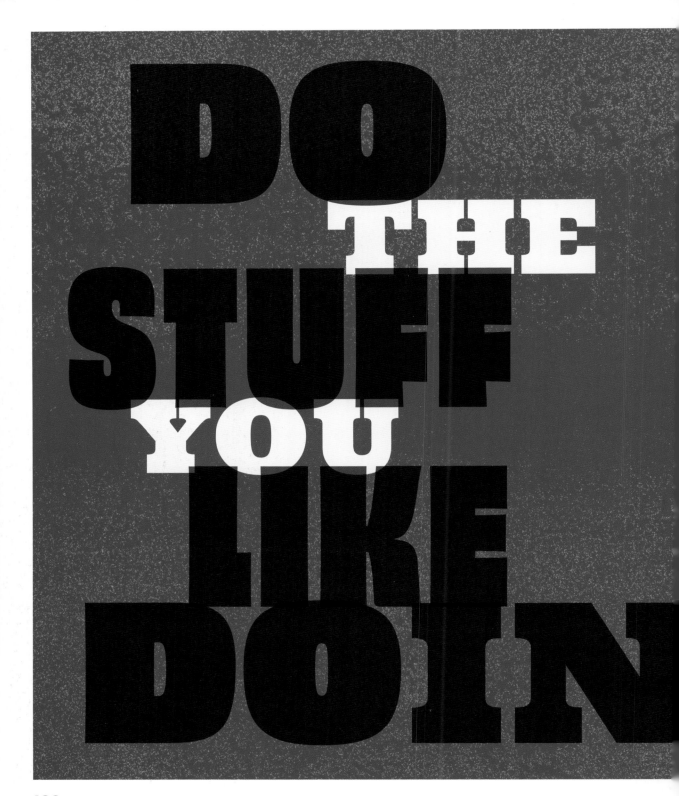

DO THE STUFF YOU LIKE DOIN

For some, cooking is high on that list.

For others, eating is even higher.

Human life can be a serious and somber affair. Of course, there are spiritual paths that offset doom and gloom, paths that I continue to travel.

But there's also things that are just plain fun.

Music.

Hanging out with friends.

Spreading love with everyone who comes your way. And eating.

Annie takes it to an art, always a crowd around our table. The simple pleasure of eating good food that you know will make your body healthier and happier.

I know this isn't the most profound thought in the world, but I believe it all the same. And every day I try to remember it:

EATING IS FUN.

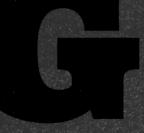

EATING MIND-FULLY

THIS MESSAGE IS TO ME:

EAT SLOWLY.

TAKE SMALL BITES.

SAVOR EACH BITE.

DON'T EAT LIKE AN ANIMAL.

FARMING

IS A

SONG

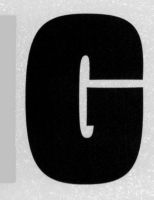

G

Farming has a vibe. Kinda like the string on a guitar after a single note bends into song. But even before the lyrics come, the vibration is a guide leading you to go deep or reach tall.

When farming, it's the vibe that tells you when a storm is coming or when the crops require special care. It's the pride that comes with an honest day's work. The satisfaction that you've done something good.

Farming is a song.

Between chores in the field and while watching the pigs play, I've gotten all sorts of musical ideas.

As a kid, I was a proud member of the Future Farmers of America, an institution that blossomed in the rural cities during the Great Depression.

Whatever responsibility and discipline I've learned, I learned it farming.

The soil is sacred. The work is noble. We started Farm Aid thirty-five years ago to honor the soil and the family farmers that work so hard to allow people to eat real food.

There are all kinds of jams.

When jazz musicians get together and play without an agenda, that's called a jam.

When country musicians jam, we call it a guitar pull or picking party.

Some folks see those as competitive battles. I don't. I see them as a loving exchange of ideas.

In the world of food, jams are also a combination of all sorts of elements jammed in a jar.

After golfing or practicing Gongkwon Yusul, a Korean mixed martial art, I'm inclined to nibble on a piece of toast with jam. When it comes to jams, though, the combinations are endless.

Here's a recipe you might find fun.

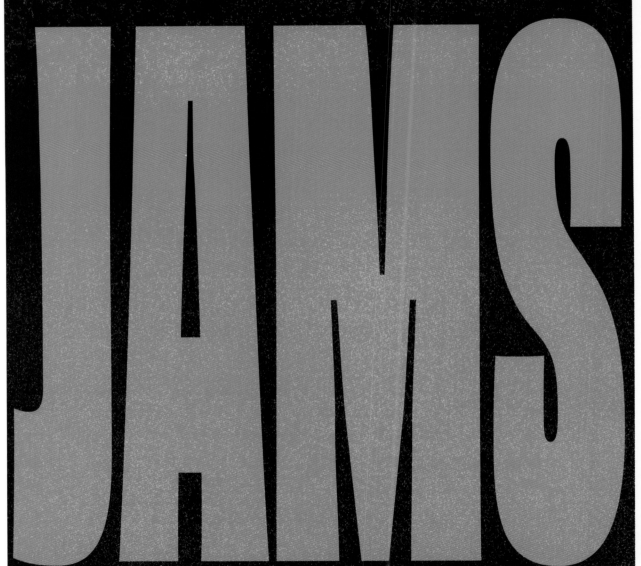

JAMS

MANDARIN MARMALADE

MAKES **6 CUPS** (96 TABLESPOONS)
7.5 MG PER SERVING (2 TABLESPOONS)

2½ pounds mandarin oranges

2 lemons

2 cups sugar

5 makrut lime leaves

6 tablespoons triple sec

1.5 grams ground Lemon Cherry Gelato cannabis 20% THC, tied in a cheesecloth sachet

Natural orange food coloring (optional)

1 Set half of the mandarins aside. Cut the remaining mandarins and the lemons in half and juice them. Yields approximately 13 to 14 fluid ounces.

2 Peel the reserved mandarins and hold on to the peels. Segment the mandarins and cut into small pieces, removing all of the seeds. This should yield roughly 1½ pounds of mandarin flesh.

3 Cut half of the reserved peels into thick strips (discard or compost the remainder). Remove the white pith from the peels by placing them pith-side up on your cutting board and using a sharp knife to slice the white portion off by laying your blade flat on the rind and cutting/slicing in the direction away from you. Alternatively you can use a vegetable peeler. It's important to remove as much of the pith as you can so that the finished product is not bitter in taste.

4 Once you've removed the pith, cut the peels into julienned slices. Set up a bowl of ice and water near the stove. Bring a small pot of water to a boil and blanch the mandarin peels for about 5 minutes. Dunk in the ice bath, drain, and set aside.

5 In a wide pot, combine the mandarin/lemon juice, mandarin flesh, blanched peel, sugar, makrut lime leaves, triple sec, and cannabis sachet. Bring to a boil for 10 minutes.

6 Reduce the heat to a simmer and cook, stirring often, for 45 minutes. The consistency should mimic a soft gel yet be fluid like honey. If it's too runny, continue to cook until you reach the desired consistency.

7 Remove from the heat, strain, and discard the cannabis sachet. The marmalade may be tinted green. If you'd like, you can add some orange food coloring. Transfer the marmalade to a glass jars and let cool at room temperature. Seal and refrigerate.

I always love writing about my friend Zeke Varnon. I'll never forget the man. I met him when I was sixteen and he was twenty-one. He was fresh out of the army and spent his evenings at the Nite Owl where my sister and I played in a band. He became my fan and I became his follower. He was a drinker and a smoker and a gambler. He taught me how to play poker, a passion that consumes me to this day.

Once we were hanging out on the porch of his home in Hillsboro, just up the road from my hometown of Abbott. It was a scorching August afternoon when one of his women friends brought by a plate piled high with thick slices of watermelon and honeydew melon.

After I started digging in, I saw that Vernon wasn't eating. I also noticed a tear in his eye.

"What's wrong?" I asked.

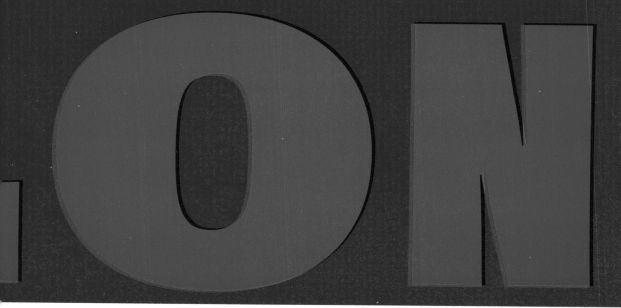

CHOLY

"Can't eat that stuff."

"Why? Couldn't be sweeter."

"It reminds me of a gal I met before I went in the service. I thought she was the one. Everything about her was right. Especially her cooking. Especially her desserts. She'd whip up fresh cream and spread it all over the watermelon. Fact is, that was the last dish she ever made for me."

"What happened?"

"She up and moved to New Orleans. Said she would find a job working in some fancy restaurant."

"And you didn't want to go with her?"

"I did but I didn't."

"And now you regret it?"

"I do when I see that food in front of me. Tasting the melon would be like tasting her. It's a taste I don't want to remember. But, man, it's a taste I'll never forget."

ON

WATERMELON RASPBERRY PRESERVES

MAKES **6 CUPS** (96 TABLESPOONS)
7.5 MG PER SERVING (2 TABLESPOONS)

6 cups coarsely grated watermelon rind (see Note)

1.5 grams ground Watermelon Zkittlez 24% THC tied in a cheesecloth sachet

3 lemons, sliced into rounds and seeded

3 tablespoons julienned fresh ginger

6 ounces raspberries

2½ teaspoons raspberry extract

5 cups baker's or superfine sugar

CHEF'S NOTE: How to achieve grated watermelon rind: Using a vegetable peeler, remove the green outer rind from the watermelon. Cut the watermelon into wedges and remove the edible flesh. Save the flesh for snacking or for adding to salads. Grate the rind, or white part of the melon, using the medium-size holes on a grater.

Enjoy the preserves on toast, biscuits, or a PB&J. It can also be used to make salad dressing.

1 Place the watermelon rind into a medium-sized bowl. Add the cannabis sachet, lemon slices, and ginger. Cover and refrigerate overnight.

2 Transfer the mixture to a pot and set over medium-high heat. Add the raspberries, raspberry extract, sugar, and 4 cups water. Stir until the sugar completely dissolves. Reduce the temperature to low heat and cook until the watermelon is supple and a light syrup forms, about 1 hour.

3 Remove and discard the cannabis sachet.

4 Spoon the preserves into sterilized canning jars. Seal the jars and process in boiling water for 10 minutes. The water line should be enough to cover the lids of the jars.

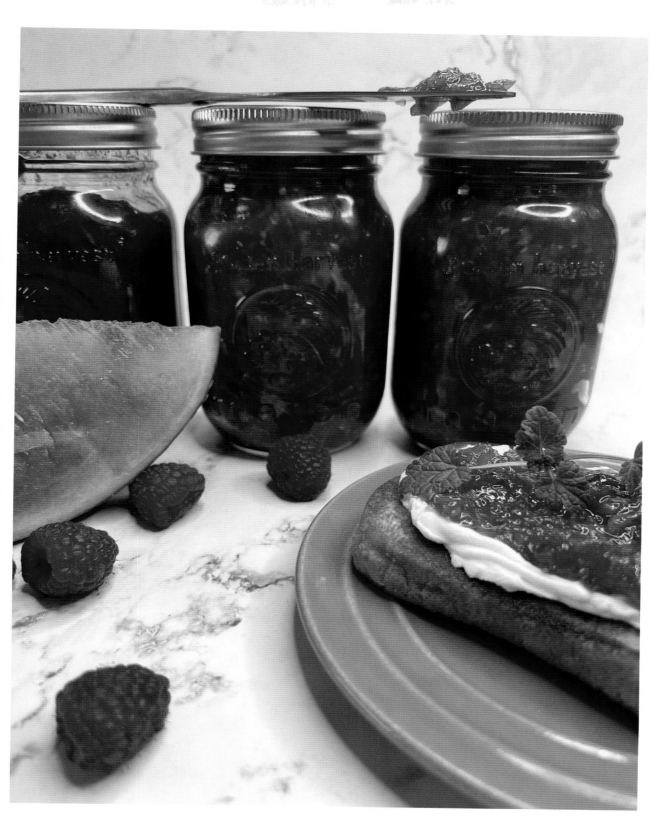

WE ARE WHAT WE EAT

>> Who can argue with that?

The food we eat does more than fill our stomachs; it supports our emotions; it either impedes or improves our spiritual and physical health.

I want to know where my food comes from.

I want to buy local.

I want to promote organic and sustainable products.

Native American practices demand that animals be killed with respect and gratitude—that their lives be revered for having given us sustenance.

This entire eating process—this cycle of refueling our energy—can be realized with or without thought.

I want to be thoughtful.

I want to remember that every time I eat anything—a pear or a pumpkin pie—I try to remember that every particle on this planet is a miracle.

SPICY CARAMBOLA FRUIT & PRAWN SALAD

MAKES **2 SERVINGS**
5.6 MG PER SERVING
(ADD **11.7 MG** PER SERVING IF USING
CANNABIS GRAPESEED OIL)

DRESSING

2 tablespoons soy sauce

2 tablespoons fresh lime juice

2 tablespoons Cannabis-Infused Simple Syrup (page 213)

2 to 3 tablespoons chili paste, to taste

1 tablespoon fish sauce

1 teaspoon red pepper flakes

1 tablespoon minced garlic

1 tablespoon toasted sesame oil

½ teaspoon Cannabis Grapeseed Oil (optional; page 11)

SALAD

5 starfruit (carambola)

8 large head-on prawns, or extra large shrimp

Kosher salt

½ red onion, thinly sliced

1 cup cherry tomatoes, halved

4 tablespoons fresh mint leaves, julienned

1 cup arugula

¼ cup cashew pieces

1 tablespoon black sesame seeds, for garnish

1 MAKE THE DRESSING: In a large bowl, whisk together the soy sauce, lime juice, simple syrup, chili paste, fish sauce, pepper flakes, and garlic until well combined. While constantly whisking, slowly drizzle in the sesame oil and cannabis oil (if using).

2 MAKE THE SALAD: Cut the starfruit lengthwise and remove the seeds. Next, cut the fruit into thin slices. Set aside.

3 Lightly season the prawns with kosher salt. Using a small amount of olive oil, grill or pan sear until cooked through, about 1 minute per side. Remove from the heat and set aside.

4 Add the starfruit and the grilled shrimp to the bowl with the salad dressing along with the onion, tomatoes, mint, arugula, and cashews and toss.

5 Split the salad between two bowls and garnish with black sesame seeds.

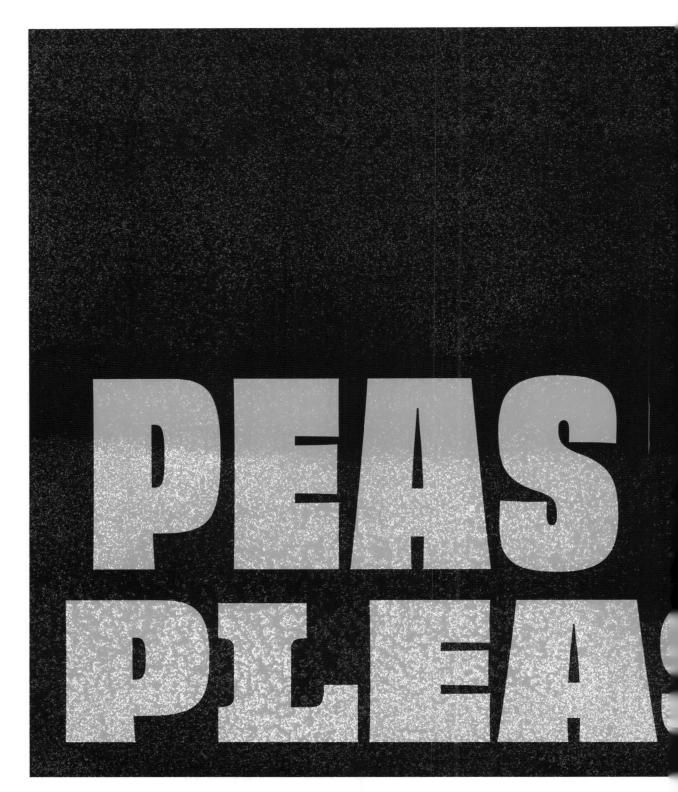

PEAS
PLEAS

1939

1939 was a rough year. My grandfather, a mighty man who made his living as a blacksmith, caught pneumonia and died at age fifty-six; I was six. That meant my grandmother, Mama Nelson, was our sole provider. But she didn't see it that way.

"God provides," was her fervent belief.

The proof was our garden.

In those lean years, our garden was our sustenance. And it was Mama Nelson who taught us to cultivate the garden, just as it was Mama Nelson who taught us to cultivate our faith.

Among other vegetables, we grew corn, tomatoes, lettuce, and black-eyed peas. The peas have a special place in my heart.

That's because on New Year's Day, 1940, Mama Nelson served up a plate of black-eyed peas.

"These peas are tradition," she told me and sister Bobbie. "They bring good fortune. I know you children are going to have good fortune in your lives. I know that because I know your hearts. Your hearts are filled with love and it's love that creates good fortune. So bless these peas and bless our household."

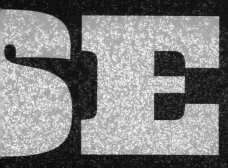

SPICY BLACK-EYED PEA HUMMUS

MAKES **4 SERVINGS**
15.8 MG PER SERVING

HUMMUS

1½ cups dried black-eyed peas

3 garlic cloves, peeled but whole

½ teaspoon tahini

½ tablespoon Tony Chachere's Creole Seasoning

2 tablespoons Cannabis Avocado Oil (page 10) or Cannabis Grapeseed Oil (page 11)

Juice of 1 lemon

½ teaspoon liquid smoke

⅓ Scotch bonnet or habañero pepper, seeded

3 to 4 ice cubes

Kosher salt

Paprika or chili powder, for dusting

GARNISH

1 tablespoon olive oil, plus more (optional) for drizzling

3 tablespoons finely diced red bell pepper

2 garlic cloves, minced

Salt

1 tablespoon fresh thyme leaves, minced

1 In a bowl, combine the black-eyed peas with water to cover and soak overnight.

2 Drain the peas and cook in a pot of boiling water until tender, 1 to 2 hours.

3 MAKE THE GARNISH: In a small skillet, heat 1 tablespoon olive oil over medium-low heat. . Add the bell pepper and minced garlic and cook until fragrant. Add 2 tablespoons of the black-eyed peas and sauté for an additional 1 to 2 minutes.

4 Remove from the heat and season with a pinch of salt. Fold in the minced thyme and set the garnish aside.

5 MAKE THE HUMMUS: In a food processor, gently pulse the remaining black-eyed peas for a few seconds. Add the whole garlic, tahini, Creole seasoning, cannabis oil, lemon juice, liquid smoke, and Scotch bonnet pepper. Pulse again for an added few seconds.

6 Add 2 ice cubes and continue to pulse until the blend is smooth and creamy. The ice cubes aid in the process of achieving the perfect smoothness. Add an additional cube, if needed. Season with salt to taste.

7 Serve the hummus topped with the garnish. Dust with paprika or chili powder. If desired, add a drizzle of olive oil.

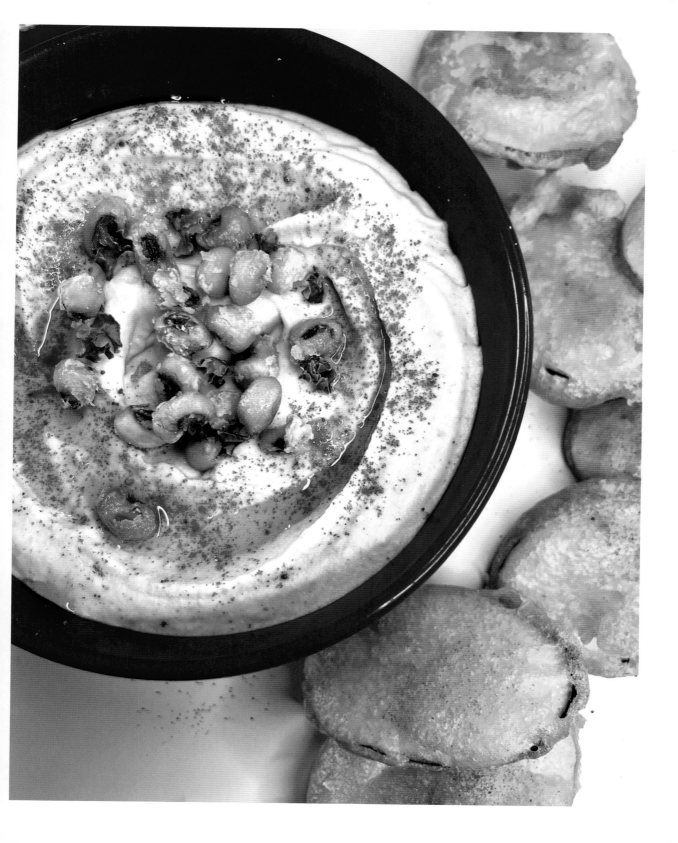

BUTTERY BEANS

Beans made right are hard to beat. Here's a different way to try it.

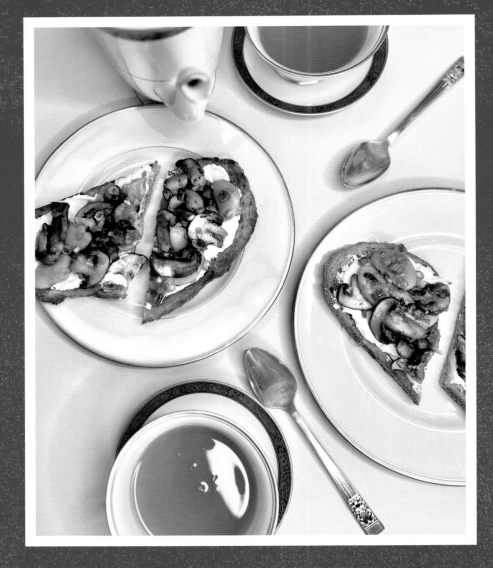

BROWNED BUTTER BUTTER BEAN TOAST WITH WHIPPED FETA

MAKES **2 SERVINGS**
29.3 MG PER SERVING (SEE NOTE)

WHIPPED FETA

- 3-ounce block feta cheese, drained
- 4 tablespoons whole Greek yogurt
- 2 teaspoons grated lemon zest
- 1 teaspoon extra-virgin olive oil
- ½ teaspoon Cannabis Avocado Oil (page 10)
- Pinch of kosher salt
- Pinch of freshly ground black pepper
- 1 teaspoon chopped fresh mint
- 1 teaspoon chopped fresh parsley

BUTTER BEAN TOAST

- 2 tablespoons butter
- ½ teaspoon Cannabis Ghee (page 9)
- 5 garlic cloves, minced
- Olive oil
- 4 large cremini mushrooms, sliced
- 1½ cups or 1 (15- ounce) can cooked butter beans
- 1 scallion, chopped
- 2 slices artisan bread, toasted

CHEF'S NOTE: The whipped feta has 11.7 mg THC per serving. The brown butter mixture has 17.6 mg THC. You can omit either or reduce the dosage using less oil or ghee.

1 MAKE THE WHIPPED FETA: In a food processor, combine the feta, Greek yogurt, and lemon zest and blend.

2 In a small bowl, combine extra-virgin olive oil and cannabis oil. With the processor running, drizzle in the oil mixture until the feta is whipped to a smooth texture.

3 Transfer to a bowl and stir in the kosher salt, black pepper, mint, and parsley. Refrigerate until ready to serve.

4 PREPARE THE TOASTS: In a heavy-bottomed skillet, melt the butter and cannabis ghee over medium heat. Whisk frequently as the butter continues to cook. The butter will foam up a bit. Lightly browned specks will begin to form and the aroma will become nutty.

5 Reduce the heat and add the minced garlic. Stir for several seconds until the garlic becomes aromatic and remove the skillet from the heat.

6 In a separate skillet, heat a splash olive oil over medium heat. Add the mushrooms and cook until golden. Add the butter beans and cook until warmed through.

7 Transfer the mixture to the brown butter and garlic blend. Add the scallion and fold in until well incorporated.

8 To serve, divide the whipped feta evenly between the two slices of toast. Top with equal portions of the butter bean mixture.

JOHNNY CASH HAD FAITH

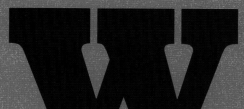

When you're broke, sometimes all you have is faith.

My first song to make me a little money was called "Family Bible." It was a song born out of faith. Fortunately, it got recorded not only by me, but by many other artists. It became a standard.

In 1998, many decades after I wrote "Family Bible," the VHI *Storytellers* show invited me and Johnny Cash. In the green room, Johnny got to talking about family and the importance of family dinners. Johnny was a man of God who believed that family dinners were occasions to renew our faith.

When it came time for us to go out before the cameras and sing, we still hadn't picked a song.

"What about the tune you wrote about a dad reading the Bible after a big family dinner?"

"You mean 'Family Bible'?" I asked.

"That's the one. Teach me the lyrics right quick."

I did, and that's the song Johnny and I sang.

When I was through, I saw a tear in Johnny's eye. He just nodded.

I believe it was the last time he and I sang together.

It's been a few years now since Johnny has passed on and rarely do I sit down to a family dinner without thinking of singing "Family Bible" with Johnny. Here's a cozy mac and cheese recipe that will warm your soul.

TRUFFLE MAC & CHEESE

MAKES **4 SERVINGS**
17.6 MG PER SERVING

4 cups whole milk

¼ onion

2 garlic cloves, peeled but whole

1 bay leaf

10½ tablespoons (5.25 ounces) butter

1 teaspoon Cannabis Ghee (page 9)

⅔ cup all-purpose flour

⅔ cup grated Comté cheese

⅔ cup grated Cheddar cheese, grated

8 ounces Urbani Black Truffles & Mushrooms (approximately 2 cans)

Kosher salt and freshly ground black pepper

2 cups uncooked macaroni

1¼ cups torn mozzarella cheese

2 tablespoons grated parmesan cheese

¼ cup grated fresh black truffle

1 tablespoon finely chopped fresh parsley

1 In a saucepan, bring the milk to just shy of a boil over medium-high heat. Add the onion, garlic cloves, and bay leaf. Remove from the heat, cover, and set aside to infuse for 30 minutes. Strain out the aromatics and discard.

2 Preheat the oven to 400°F.

3 In another saucepan, melt the butter and cannabis ghee over low heat. Whisk in the flour to create a roux. Cook for 1 minute while continuing to whisk. Gradually whisk in the warm infused milk until the mixture is smooth. Slowly bring to a boil over low heat, whisking constantly until the sauce thickens. Simmer gently for 5 minutes, stirring often.

4 Add the Comté and cheddar and whisk in until smooth. Add the Urbani truffles & mushrooms and stir until fully incorporated. Season to taste with salt and pepper.

5 Meanwhile, in a large pan of salted boiling water, cook the macaroni to al dente according to the package directions. Drain and cool under cold running water and drain again.

6 Add the drained macaroni to the cheese sauce and mix well to coat. Pour the mixture into a 2 quart gratin dish. Scatter the mozzarella on top, and sprinkle with the parmesan.

7 Bake until the topping is golden, 15 to 20 minutes.

8 Shave the black truffle on top, garnish with chopped parsley, and serve.

TUSCAN RABBIT

MAKES **3 SERVINGS**
15.6 MG PER SERVING

2 tablespoons all-purpose flour

Kosher salt and freshly ground black pepper

1 whole rabbit, butcher cut

3 tablespoons olive oil (add more if needed)

1 teaspoon Cannabis Grapeseed Oil (page 11)

1 teaspoon fennel seeds

2 onions, finely chopped

6 slices bacon, chopped

4 garlic cloves, minced

1 cup white wine

⅓ cup balsamic vinegar

1¾ cups diced canned tomatoes

1¾ cups cherry tomatoes

2 sprigs fresh rosemary, leaves picked and minced

2 tablespoons chopped fresh flat-leaf parsley

CHEF'S NOTE: Serve with creamy polenta.

1 Preheat the oven to 350°F.

2 In a small bowl, season the flour with salt and pepper. Dust the rabbit pieces in the seasoned flour, shaking off any excess.

3 In a skillet, heat 2 tablespoons of the olive oil over medium heat, Working in batches, add the rabbit and cook until golden, about 2 minutes per side. Transfer to a baking dish.

4 In the same skillet, heat the remaining 1 tablespoon olive oil and the cannabis oil over medium heat. Add the fennel, onions, bacon, and garlic and cook, stirring, until soft and golden, 3 to 4 minutes. Add the wine and half the vinegar and simmer for 3 to 4 minutes to reduce by half.

5 Add the canned tomatoes, cherry tomatoes, and rosemary. Season with salt and pepper and bring to a boil.

6 Pour the tomato mixture over the rabbit. Cover the baking dish, transfer to the oven, and cook until the rabbit is tender, 1 hour 15 minutes.

7 Stir in the remaining vinegar and finish with chopped parsley.

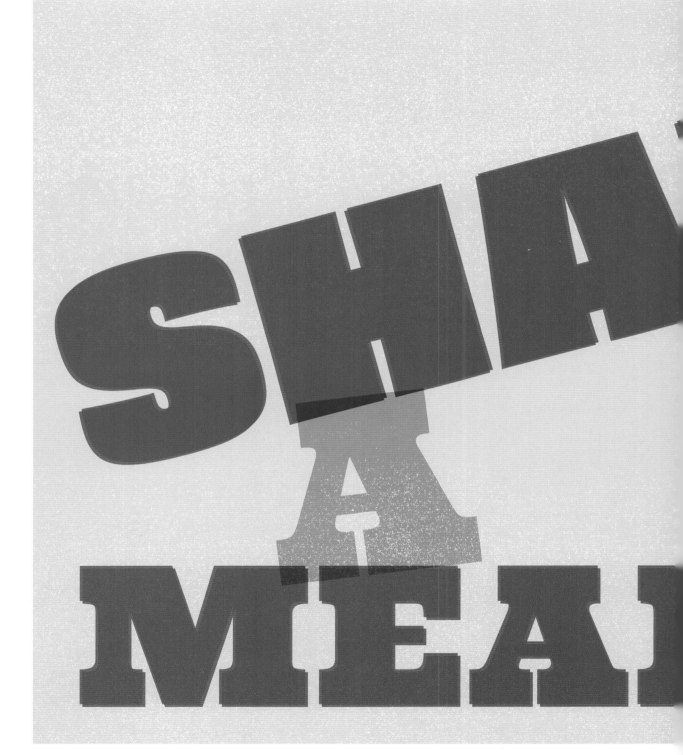

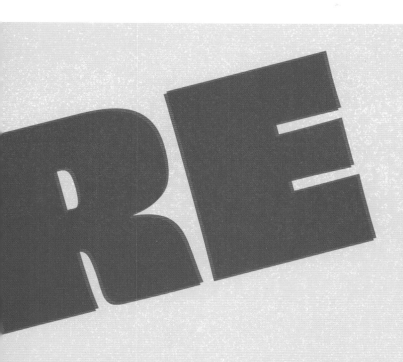

Getting together for a satisfying meal is a good time to put down technology and to catch up with family and friends. A good time to get off the grid and get a grip on what fellowship is all about. Sharing a meal is a sacred ritual and to Annie, a shared meal is shared love.

Creating a meal is more than throwing together some ingredients. It's artful. It's about preparing something delicious with tender loving care. It's one of the most moving and beautiful things we human beings can do together.

At mealtime, we lean in and listen to each other. We learn. We express empathy. We encourage.

THE SENSU

THE SENSU

"TO UNDERSTAND A WOMAN'S SENSUALITY, WATCH HOW SHE EATS."
—FEDERICO FELLINI

Guess you could say the same of a man. Either way, it's not a bad observation. Food is sensual. According to my handy dictionary, sensual has to do with gratifying the senses or indulging physical appetites.

I like gratification. I like making my mouth happy. I like getting my tongue involved. I believe it's healthy to look at food as an instrument of pure pleasure.

When it comes to food sensuality, I think of fruit. Sweet grapes. Tart apples. Ripe avocados. Slice open a juicy peach or a fig. Get down with a mess of mangoes.

A sensual relationship with the right dish can do wonders for the spirit.

Try out this newfangled fruit concoction that you can savor morning, noon, or night.

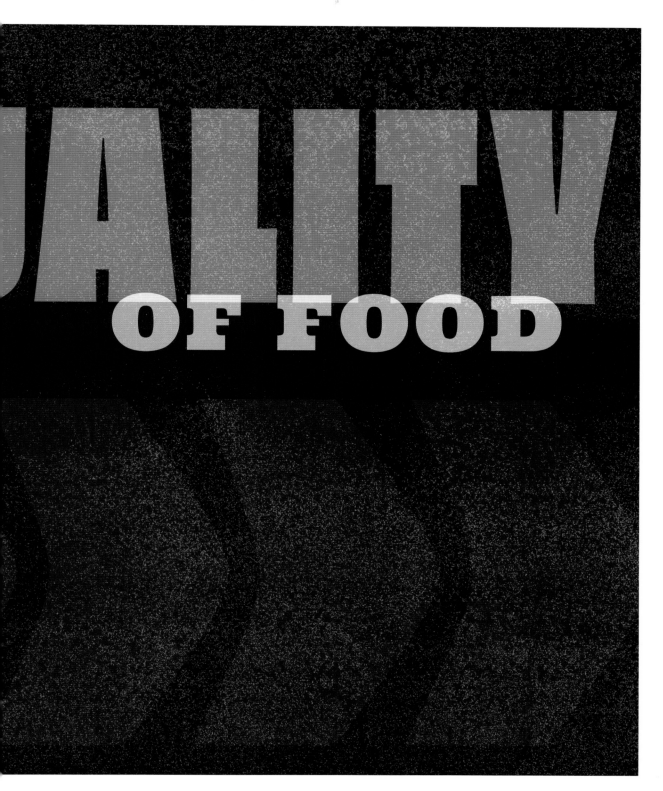

QUALITY OF FOOD

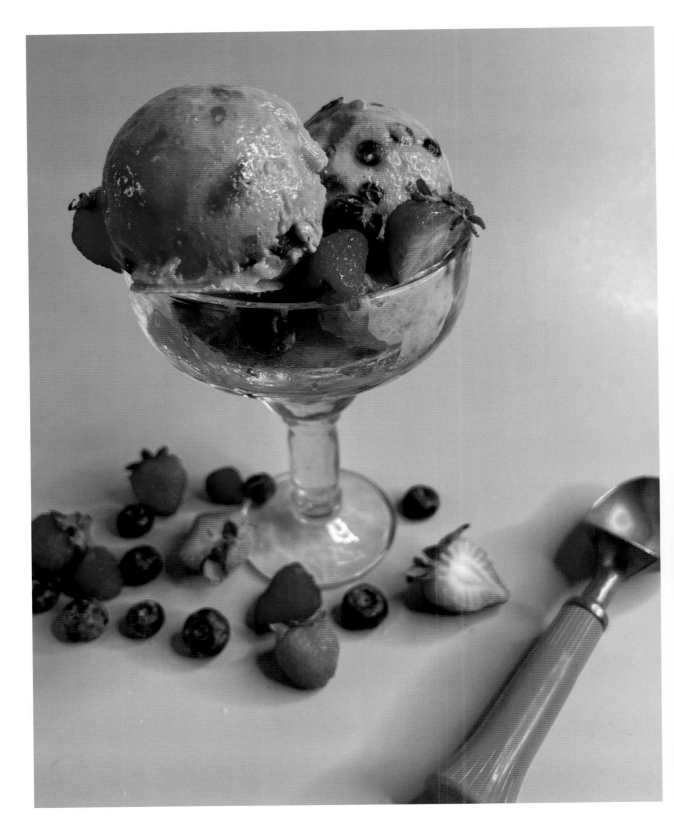

MIXED-BERRY VEGAN ICE CREAM

MAKES **6 SERVINGS**
7.5 MG PER SERVING

4 cups frozen mixed berries
1 cup full-fat coconut milk
½ cup Cannabis-Infused
   Simple Syrup (page 213)

In a food processor, combine the frozen berries, coconut milk, and cannabis simple syrup and process until smooth. Transfer to a freezer-safe container and place in the freezer for 2 hours. Stir occasionally for a smoother ice cream texture.

WATERMELON GRANITA WITH SWEET BASIL PESTO

MAKES **6 SERVINGS**
12.8 MG PER SERVING
(SUBTRACT **7.8 MG** IF NOT SERVING
WITH THE PESTO)

GRANITA

1½ pounds watermelon flesh, chopped and seeded

⅓ cup Cannabis-Infused Simple Syrup (recipe follows)

2 tablespoons fresh lemon juice

¼ teaspoon kosher salt

SWEET BASIL PESTO

1 cup fresh basil leaves

1 cup fresh mint leaves

⅓ cup grapeseed oil

3 tablespoons olive oil

1 teaspoon Cannabis Grapeseed Oil (page 11)

⅓ cup pine nuts

3 tablespoons raw honey

1 vanilla bean pod, split lengthwise, or 1 teaspoon vanilla extract

1 MAKE THE GRANITA: In a blender, combine the watermelon, cannabis simple syrup, lemon juice, and salt and blend until smooth. Strain the mixture through a fine-mesh sieve. Transfer the strained mixture to a freezer-safe baking dish. Freeze for at least 4 hours, scraping with a fork every 40 minutes to create small ice crystals.

2 MEANWHILE, MAKE THE SWEET BASIL PESTO: In a food processor, combine the basil, mint, grapeseed oil, olive oil, cannabis oil, pine nuts, and honey. Scrape the seeds from the vanilla bean into the food processor (or add the vanilla extract). Blend until smooth.

3 To serve, divide the granita among six bowls and top each with 3 tablespoons of sweet pesto.

CHEF'S NOTE: If you're up for the extra task, serve this with freshly whipped cream.

CANNABIS-INFUSED SIMPLE SYRUP

MAKES **4 CUPS** (64 TABLESPOONS)
90 MG PER CUP (5.6 MG PER TABLESPOON)

3 cups sugar

1.5 grams ground Watermelon Zkittlez cannabis, tied in a cheesecloth sachet

1 In a medium saucepan, combine the sugar and 3 cups water and bring to a boil over medium heat.

2 Add the ground cannabis cachet, reduce the heat, and stir until the sugar dissolves. Cover and allow the syrup to simmer over low heat for 20 minutes.

3 Remove from the heat and allow it to cool. Discard the sachet. Keep the simple syrup in the refrigerator.

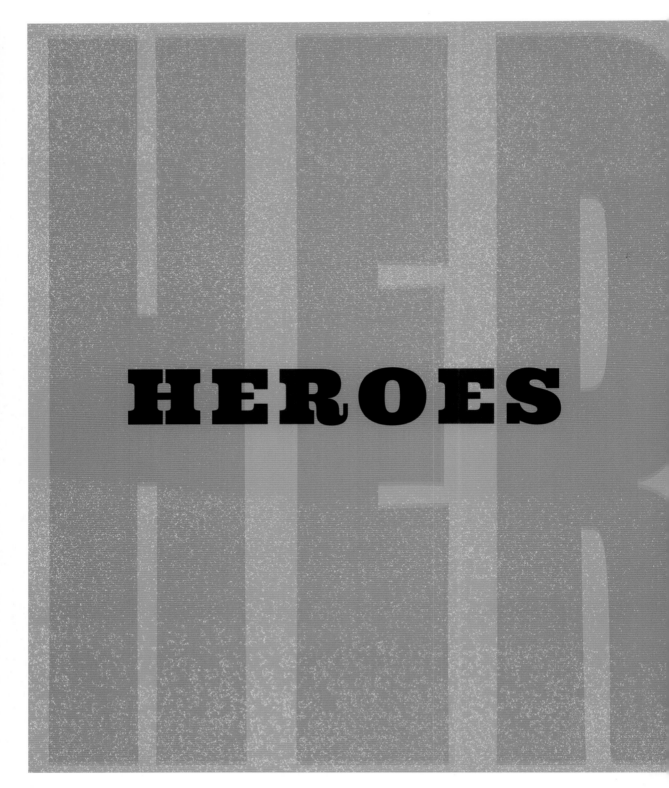

HEROES

The prairie is vast. The air is still. In the distance, coyotes howl at a crescent moon. The fire crackles. The cowboy prepares his chow.

The cowboy could be Gene Autry, Roy Rogers, Wild Bill Elliot, or Hopalong Cassidy.

These were the heroes of my childhood as I sat in a movie theater in Hillsboro, Texas, watching them cook the kind of food that, in my ten-year-old imagination, real men ate.

Beyond the most obvious qualities that I admire about these cowboys—their bravery, their sense of morality, their quickness on the draw—I also got the message that cooking wasn't only for women. Men knew how to make do in the great outdoors. They could make a stew, they could scramble eggs, and they could brew coffee.

Sometimes my mind goes back to Lash LaRue or Whip Wilson having their breakfast as the sun rises over a landscape of Arizona cacti.

Kitchens are beautiful. They come in all shapes and sizes. They contain endless assortments of wondrous instruments for preparing wondrous meals.

But there's something about cooking in the great outdoors. The great outdoors can be a tiny backyard in a big city or a 100-acre ranch. Doesn't matter. What matters is the smoke curling up in the sky, the delicious aroma, the feeling of freedom.

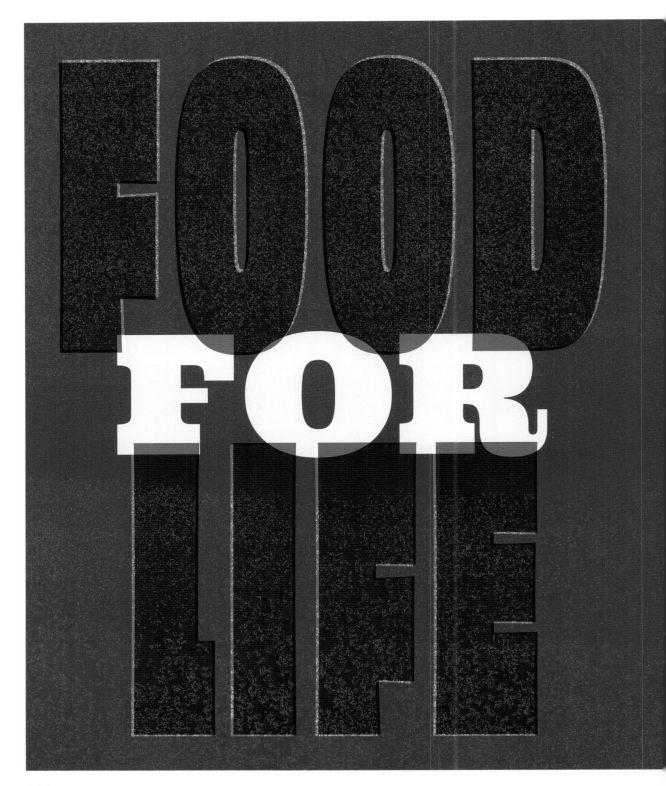

FOOD FOR LIFE

I wrote a song about how I don't go to funerals, and I won't be at mine. A dear friend of mine died. This special human being meant so much to me. I knew his death was imminent, but when it happened it still hit me like a ton of bricks. I was like the walking wounded.

Even though I didn't go to the funeral, I did come by to pay my respects to the family the next day. I sat with the bereaved relatives in silence. The silence was riddled with pain. At one point the door opened and a friend carried in a plate of vegetables she had just picked from the garden. The lettuce was green and the tomatoes were as red as the sun. I know it sounds strange, but it was almost as though the carrots and cucumbers and peas and beans were singing to me. The song said, "Pain is real, death is real, but here is new life. Life doesn't end."

Fresh foods remind me that life is all around us.

MISO CAESAR SALAD

MAKES **6 SERVINGS**
23.5 MG PER SERVING

1 cup small cubes sourdough bread

2 tablespoons toasted sesame oil

Kosher salt

½ cup Homemade Mayonnaise (recipe follows)

¼ cup white miso

1 tablespoon olive oil

1 tablespoon Cannabis Avocado Oil (page 10)

2 garlic cloves, finely chopped

2 white anchovy fillets, finely chopped

1 teaspoon white wine vinegar

½ teaspoon freshly ground black pepper

¼ teaspoon Worcestershire sauce

8 cups shredded lacinato kale leaves (stems and midribs removed)

1 tablespoon black sesame seeds

1 tablespoon hemp hearts

1 medium avocado, cubed

1½ cups half-moons peeled daikon radish

1 Preheat the oven to 350°F.

2 Drizzle the cubed sourdough bread with the sesame oil and lightly season with kosher salt. Toss to evenly coat the cubed bread.

3 Arrange on a baking sheet and bake until the croutons are golden and crispy, 5 to 7 minutes. Set aside to cool.

4 In a large bowl, whisk together the chilled homemade mayonnaise, white miso, olive oil, cannabis oil, garlic, anchovies, white wine vinegar, pepper, Worcestershire, and 3 tablespoons water. Add the shredded kale, sesame seeds, hemp hearts, cubed avocado, daikon radish, and sesame croutons. Gently toss together. Serve immediately.

HOMEMADE MAYONNAISE

MAKES 1 CUP

1 large egg, at room
  temperature
1 tablespoon Dijon
  mustard
1 tablespoon red
  wine vinegar, plus
  more to taste
¼ teaspoon kosher
  salt, plus more to
  taste
1 cup grapeseed oil
1 teaspoon fresh
  lemon juice, plus
  more to taste

1 In a small food processor, process the egg for 20 seconds. Add the mustard, vinegar, and salt and process for another 20 seconds.

2 Scrape the sides and bottom of the bowl. Continue to mix while slowly adding ¼ cup of the oil into the processor in drops. When the mixture is beginning to thicken and emulsify, continue to add the remainder of the oil slowly, but increase to a very thin stream instead of drops of oil.

3 Scrape the bottom and sides of the bowl and process for an extra 10 seconds. Adjust seasoning by adding more salt, lemon juice, or vinegar. If the mayo seems too thin, slowly stream in more oil with the processor running until thick. Refrigerate for at least 1 hour before using.

ROASTED BEET & PEAR SALAD WITH APRICOT DRESSING

MAKES **4 SERVINGS**
11.5 MG PER SERVING

2 fresh apricots, chopped

2 tablespoons apple cider vinegar

1 tablespoon honey

1 teaspoon Dijon mustard

¼ teaspoon kosher salt

¼ teaspoon freshly ground black pepper

¼ cup extra-virgin olive oil

1 teaspoon Cannabis Avocado Oil (page 10)

3 cups mixed greens

¼ cup fresh mint leaves

½ cup chopped radicchio

3 medium roasted beets, cubed (pre-packaged optional)

1 ripe pear, diced

¼ cup pistachios

½ cup thinly sliced red onion

¼ cup crumbled feta cheese

1 In a blender, combine the apricots, vinegar, honey, mustard, salt, and black pepper and puree until smooth.

2 In a spouted measuring cup, stir the olive oil and cannabis oil together. With the blender is running on low speed, slowly drizzle in the oil mixture until well incorporated into a salad dressing consistency. Adjust seasoning to taste.

3 In a large bowl, combine the mixed greens, mint, and radicchio. Add the salad dressing and toss to coat evenly.

4 Divide the greens among four plates. Dividing evenly, top with beets, pear, pistachios, red onion, and feta.

LETTUCE

&

We loved in springtime
When the world was new
A season of sunshine
Our troubles were few
Flowers blooming
Gardens fresh and green
But not everything
Was quite what it seemed

That's the start of a song I never finished. Like a lot of my love songs, it was heading for an unhappy ending, so I figured I'd leave the happy couple alone—at least for a while—and let the good feelings linger.

I have a good feeling for lettuce. Iceberg. Romaine. Butter. I love tomatoes. Love cucumbers and onions. Love anything that takes me back to the garden of my childhood.

You can look at life like one big salad.

LOVE

ALL PRAISES TO THE GREEN G

The older I get, the more I'm into health food. I credit my wife, Annie, a tireless champion of organic products.

On the road, finding fresh food isn't easy. But Annie is resourceful using the Internet to identify farmers' markets and health food stores along the way.

I don't like playing on a full stomach, but I do need energy to perform. That's why protein drinks serve me so well.

I especially love the Green Goddess smoothie. It's packed full of vegetables that satisfy my hunger—plus I don't feel bloated.

Here's a customized Green Goddess certain to boost your energy and help you beat back the midday blues.

ODDESS

GREEN SMOOTHIE BOWLS

MAKES **2 SERVINGS**
5.6 MG PER SERVING

SMOOTHIE

1 cup frozen banana slices

2 tablespoons Cannabis-Infused Simple Syrup (page 213)

2 cups frozen pineapple

2 cups spinach

2 scoops Athletic Greens AG1 supplement (optional)

7 ounces full-fat coconut milk

BOWLS

2 tablespoons hemp hearts

1 kiwi, peeled and sliced

3 tablespoons blackberries

2 tablespoons pomegranate seeds

1 MAKE THE SMOOTHIES: In a blender, combine all the ingredients except the coconut milk. Blend on low or pulse. Move the fruit around if necessary.

2 Add the coconut milk in small increments and blend. Continue this process until you achieve the smoothness and thickness desired.

3 ASSEMBLE THE BOWLS: Divide the smoothie between two bowls. Top with hemp hearts, kiwi, blackberries, and pomegranate seeds.

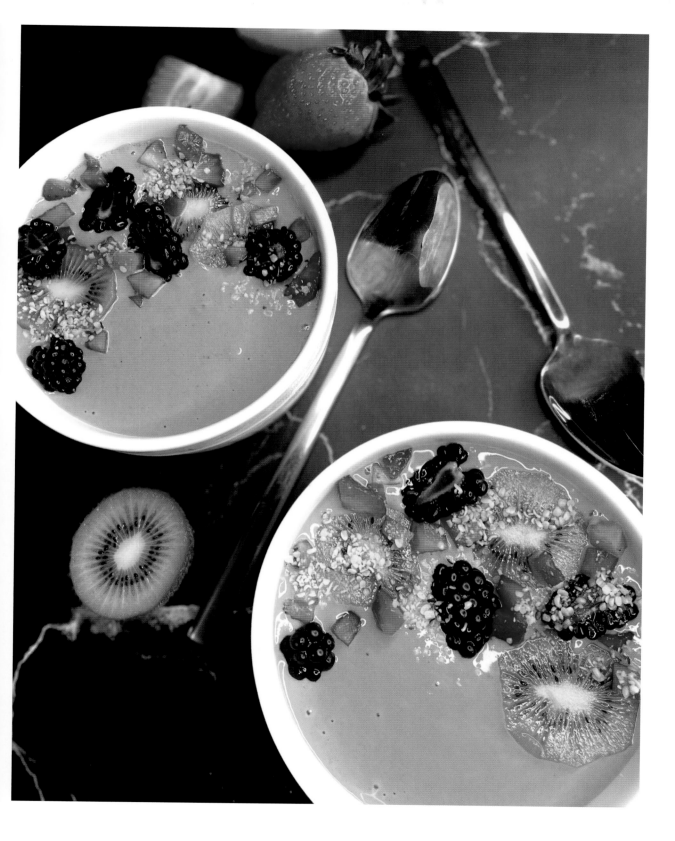

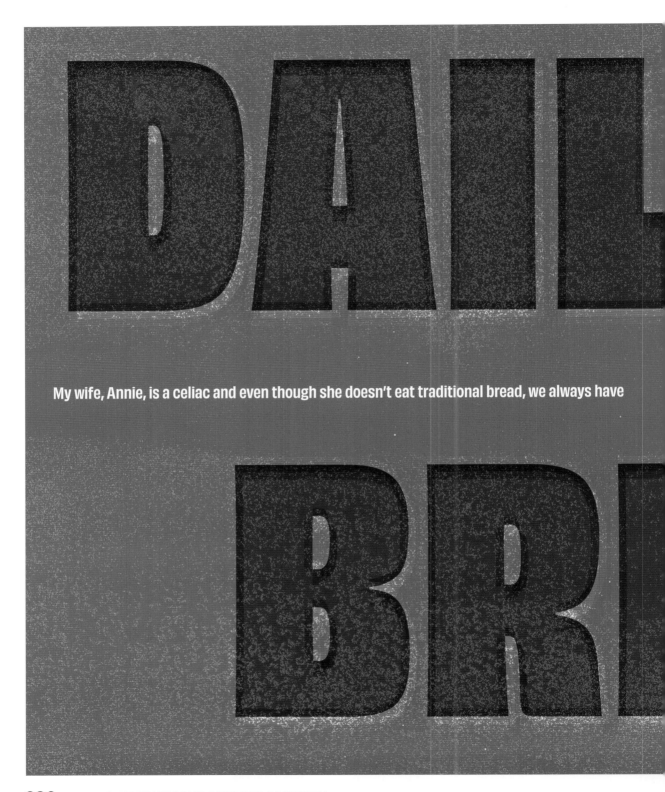

DAIL BRE

My wife, Annie, is a celiac and even though she doesn't eat traditional bread, we always have

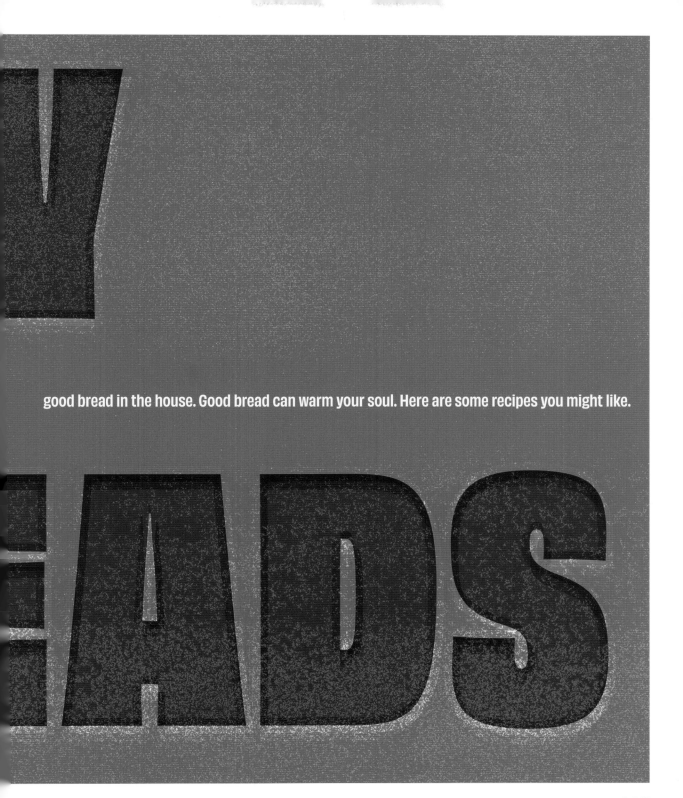

good bread in the house. Good bread can warm your soul. Here are some recipes you might like.

CORNBREAD BRIOCHE BUNS

MAKES **9 ROLLS**
13.4 MG PER ROLL

4½ teaspoons instant yeast

2½ cups bread flour, plus more as needed

1 cup cornmeal

2 tablespoons sugar

1 tablespoon kosher salt

1½ tablespoons blackstrap molasses

7 tablespoons (3½ ounces) butter, diced, at room temperature, plus more for the bowl

1 tablespoon Cannabis Ghee (page 9)

1 large egg

Cooking spray

Egg wash: 1 egg, whisked well

Black sesame seeds

CHEF'S NOTE: Serve as a side or use as a bun for sandwiches.

1 In a stand mixer, whisk the yeast into 1 cup water until fully dissolved and allow to develop for 5 to 10 minutes, until it starts to bubble.

2 Add the bread flour, cornmeal, sugar, salt, molasses, butter, cannabis ghee, and egg to the bowl. Using the paddle attachment, mix for about 7 minutes until the ingredients are well incorporated and the dough is tacky. The dough should release from the bottom of the bowl. Add additional flour if needed to release the dough.

3 Transfer the dough to a buttered bowl. Wrap loosely with plastic and allow it to proof until it triples in size, about 4 hours.

4 Remove the plastic wrap and punch down the dough. Divide the dough into 9 equal portions (about 4 ounces each) and roll into balls.

5 Spray a baking pan that can fit all of the rolls, but leave enough space between them to triple in size. Add the rolls to the pan, wrap loosely with plastic, and again allow to proof for up to an hour.

6 Meanwhile, preheat the oven to 350°F.

7 Gently brush the tops of the buns with the egg wash. Proceed with caution so as not to deflate the buns. Top with black sesame seeds.

8 Bake until the buns are a deep golden brown, about 20 minutes, rotating the pan front to back halfway through.

9 Remove from the oven and allow to cool in the pan.

SOUTHERN HOE CAKES WITH CALABRIAN HONEY BUTTER

MAKES **8 CAKES**
5.8 MG PER SERVING
(ADD **14.2 MG** PER SERVING IF USING
CALABRIAN HONEY BUTTER)

- 1 cup finely ground yellow cornmeal
- 2 tablespoons sweet corn powder
- 1 cup all-purpose flour
- 2 tablespoons sugar
- 1 tablespoon baking powder
- 1 teaspoon kosher salt
- 1 cup buttermilk
- ¼ cup vegetable oil, plus more for frying
- 1 teaspoon Cannabis Coconut Oil (page 10)
- 2 large eggs
- 2 to 4 tablespoons salted or unsalted butter, for frying
- ½ cup Calabrian Honey Butter (recipe follows), for serving (1 tablespoon per cake)

1 In a medium bowl, whisk together the cornmeal, corn powder, flour, sugar, baking powder, and salt. Add the buttermilk, ¼ cup vegetable oil, cannabis coconut oil, and eggs. Whisk together until thick, creamy, and thoroughly combined.

2 In a large skillet, heat equal parts oil and butter over medium-high heat. Working in batches, add ¼ to ⅓ cup batter to form into even-size rounds. Cook until golden and puffed, about 2 minutes per side. Transfer to a platter and keep warm. Add additional oil and butter for each batch.

3 Serve hot with 1 tablespoon Calabrian honey butter per hoe cake.

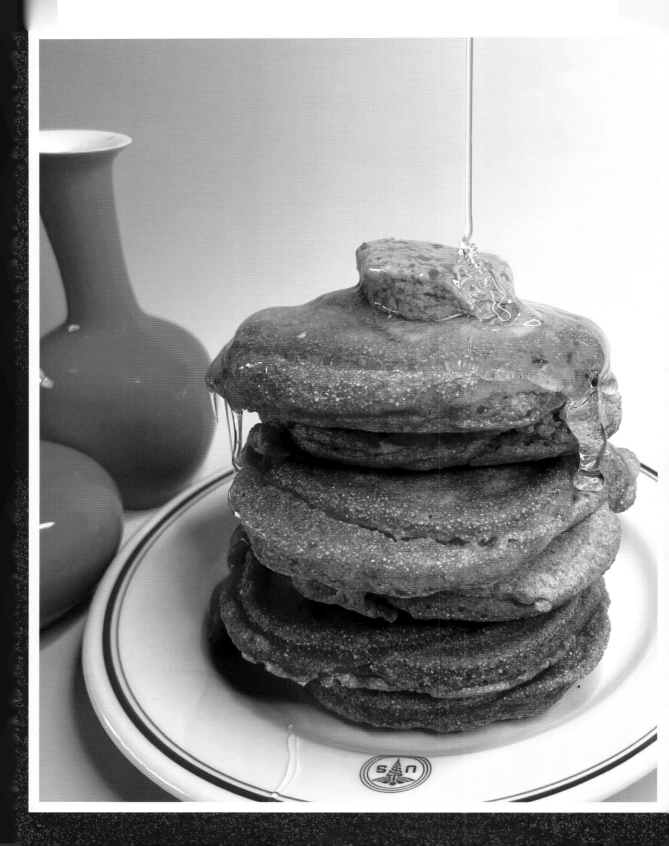

CALABRIAN HONEY BUTTER

MAKES **1 CUP**
212 MG THC
14.2 MG PER SERVING (I TABLESPOON)

14 tablespoons
    (7 ounces) butter,
    at room
    temperature
1 tablespoon Cannabis
    Ghee (page 9)
⅓ cup honey
Grated zest of 1 orange
1 teaspoon kosher salt
3 oil-packed Calabrian
    chiles, finely minced

In a bowl, whisk together the softened butter, cannabis ghee, honey, orange zest, kosher salt, and chiles until thoroughly combined and smooth. Transfer to a butter mold or ramekin and refrigerate.

SEEDED FOCACCIA

MAKES **10 SERVINGS**
NO THC
(ADD **14.1 MG** PER SERVING IF HAVING
WITH KALAMATA OLIVE BUTTER)

1 (7-gram) envelope active dry yeast (2¼ teaspoons)

2 teaspoons honey

2 teaspoons warm water

5 cups all-purpose flour

3½ teaspoons kosher salt

6 tablespoons extra-virgin olive oil, plus more for drizzling

¼ cup hemp hearts

¼ cup sunflower seeds

¼ cup black sesame seeds

6 garlic cloves, sliced or minced

2 tablespoons extra virgin olive oil

Kalamata Olive Butter (optional; recipe follows)

1 In a bowl, whisk together the yeast, honey, and water until all of the yeast dissolves. Allow it to stand for 5 minutes or until the mixture foams.

2 Add the flour and kosher salt and incorporate thoroughly using a rubber spatula.

3 Pour 5 tablespoons of the extra-virgin olive oil into a separate bowl. Transfer the dough to the bowl, turning it until the dough is fully coated with the oil. Wrap the bowl with plastic and refrigerate for 8 hours, until the dough has doubled in size.

4 Oil a 9 × 13-inch baking pan with the remaining 1 tablespoon extra-virgin olive oil. Transfer the dough to the baking pan and drizzle with olive oil to coat.

5 Cover the pan with plastic wrap and allow it to proof at room temperature until doubled in size, about 4 hours.

6 Position a rack in the center of the oven and preheat the oven to 450°F.

7 In a small bowl, combine the hemp hearts, sunflower seeds, sesame seeds, garlic, and olive oil.

8 Uncover the proofed dough and use the tips of your fingers to dimple the dough while stretching it to fit the size of the pan.

9 Evenly drizzle the garlic/seed mixture across the surface of the dimpled dough.

10 Transfer to the oven and bake until golden, 20 to 30 minutes.

11 Serve warm. If desired, have each serving with 1½ tablespoons kalamata olive butter.

KALAMATA OLIVE BUTTER

YIELDS **10 SERVINGS**
MAKES **1 CUP**
14.1 MG PER TABLESPOON

14 tablespoons salted butter, at room temperature

1 tablespoon Cannabis Ghee (page 9), at room temperature

2 teaspoons garlic-shallot puree (see Note)

2 tablespoons finely chopped fresh parsley

½ cup finely chopped pitted kalamata olives

In a bowl, thoroughly mix together the softened butter, cannabis ghee, garlic-shallot puree, parsley, and olives. Incorporate the ingredients so that there are no streaks. Roll into a log and wrap in plastic wrap or store in a ramekin. Keep in the refrigerator.

CHEF'S NOTE: to make the garlic-shallot puree:

* 10 cloves garlic, peeled

* ½ of a large shallot, peeled

* 1 tablespoon olive oil

Mix together in a mini food processor or blender for about 30 seconds. Scrape down and blend until creamy.

VEGAN HEMP HEART BUNS

MAKES **8 BUNS**
17.6 MG PER BUN

4¾ cups all-purpose flour, plus more for dusting

2 tablespoons granulated sugar

1 (7-gram) envelope instant yeast (2¼ teaspoons)

2 teaspoons sea salt

1½ cups warm water

3 tablespoons olive oil, plus more for the bowl

1 tablespoon Cannabis Grapeseed Oil (page 11)

3 tablespoons unsweetened oat milk

1 teaspoon agave syrup

1 teaspoon Dijon mustard

1 tablespoon hemp hearts, for topping

1 In a large bowl, whisk together the flour, sugar, yeast, and salt. Create a well in the center of the dry ingredients and slowly pour in the warm water, olive oil, and cannabis oil. Mix thoroughly with impeccably clean hands or spatula. The dough will appear shaggy.

2 Turn the dough out onto a flour-dusted work surface. Flour your hands and knead the dough for 8 to 10 minutes. Add additional flour if necessary (up to an additional ¼ cup for dusting). The end result should be smooth.

3 Lightly grease the dough with additional oil and transfer back to the bowl. Cover loosely with plastic wrap or a kitchen towel and let it sit in a warm area until it doubles in size, at least 1 hour. You can place it in the oven on the OFF setting to help it rise.

4 Punch down the dough and knead. Divide into 8 equal portions and roll each into a ball. Transfer the rolls to a 9 x 13-inch baking dish big enough that the rolls can sit about 4 inches apart.

5 Cover with a light kitchen towel and allow the rolls to proof for an additional 45 minutes. Meanwhile, preheat the oven to 400°F for at least 20 minutes before baking.

6 In a small bowl, stir together the milk, agave syrup, and mustard. Gently bush the tops of each roll with the milk mixture and sprinkle with hemp hearts.

7 Bake the buns until golden brown, about 15 minutes. Transfer the rolls to a wire rack to cool completely.

HERBED BUTTERMILK BISCUITS

MAKES **12 BISCUITS**
11.7 MG PER BISCUIT
(**19.2 MG** PER BISCUIT IF SERVING WITH
2 TABLESPOONS MANDARIN MARMALADE)

1 cup cold buttermilk

2 teaspoons honey, warmed

1 tablespoon Cannabis Avocado Oil (page 10) or Cannabis Grapeseed Oil (page 11)

3½ cups all-purpose flour, plus more for dusting

2½ teaspoons baking powder

2 teaspoons kosher salt

1 teaspoon minced fresh rosemary

1 teaspoon minced fresh thyme

1 teaspoon minced fresh sage

¼ teaspoon baking soda

2 sticks (8 ounces) cold unsalted butter, cut into ½-inch pieces, plus more, melted, for brushing

Mandarin Marmalade (optional; page 189), for serving

1 Preheat the oven to 425°F. Line a baking sheet with parchment paper.

2 In a bowl, mix together the buttermilk, honey, and cannabis oil. The mixture will not completely blend, but it will be fine when added to the dry ingredients.

3 In a food processor, pulse together the flour, baking powder, salt, fresh herbs, and baking soda until well combined. Add the chilled butter and pulse until the pieces of butter are the size of a pea.

4 Transfer to a large bowl and gradually drizzle the buttermilk mixture on top. Use a fork to toss and incorporate the wet mixture as you drizzle. Knead mixture a few times in the bowl until a shaggy dough forms.

5 Turn the dough out onto a clean surface and pat into a square 1 inch thick. Using a bench scraper or knife, cut the dough into 4 strips and stack them on top of each other. Slightly press down to flatten and, using the bench scraper, lift the dough and dust the surface with more flour. Roll the dough into a 1-inch thick rectangle and trim to create clean edges.

6 Cut the dough into 12 uniform biscuits. Transfer to the lined baking sheet, spacing them 2 inches apart, and freeze for 10 minutes.

7 Brush the tops of the biscuits with melted butter and transfer to the oven. Reduce the oven temperature to 400°F and bake until the biscuits are a deep golden brown on bottom and golden on top, 20 to 25 minutes.

8 Optionally, serve each biscuit with mandarin marmalade.

ORANGE MATCHA PISTACHIO STICKY BUNS

MAKES **12 BUNS**
26.5 MG PER BUN

DOUGH
2 cups bread flour, plus more for dusting

1 teaspoon active dry yeast

3 tablespoons light brown sugar

1 tablespoon matcha powder

½ teaspoon kosher salt

1 cup whole milk

5 tablespoons unsalted butter

Vegetable oil, for the bowl

FILLING
9 tablespoons (4½ ounces) butter, at room temperature

1½ tablespoons Cannabis Ghee (page 9), at room temperature

1 cup finely chopped pistachios

3 tablespoons light brown sugar

Grated zest of 2 large oranges

½ teaspoon orange extract

2 teaspoons matcha powder

2 teaspoons ground cinnamon

¼ teaspoon kosher salt

Pinch of ground allspice

FROSTING & GARNISH
3 ounces cream cheese, at room temperature

2 tablespoons unsalted butter, at room temperature

1½ teaspoons orange extract

1 teaspoon grated orange zest

2½ cups powdered sugar

Matcha powder, for dusting

Chopped pistachios, for garnish

1 MAKE THE DOUGH: In a large bowl, combine the flour, yeast, brown sugar, matcha powder, and salt.

2 In a small saucepan, heat the milk and butter over low heat, swirling the pan regularly until beginning to steam. Pour into a bowl and set aside to cool to room temperature.

3 Make a well in the dry ingredients, then pour in the cooled milk/butter mixture. Swiftly combine using a spoon, then turn out onto a floured surface and knead the dough for 10 minutes. (Alternatively, knead the dough in a stand mixer with the dough hook for 7 minutes.)

4 Transfer the dough to a lightly oiled bowl, cover, and leave in a warm place until doubled in size, at least 1 hour. (Alternatively, for the best flavor, leave the dough to rise in the fridge overnight.)

5 MEANWHILE, MAKE THE FILLING: In a bowl, beat together the butter, cannabis ghee, pistachios, brown sugar, orange zest, orange extract, matcha powder, cinnamon, salt, and allspice.

6 Tip the dough onto a lightly floured surface, shape into a rough rectangle, then roll out until it's about 18 × 14 inches. Spread the cinnamon/pistachio butter over the dough, all the way out to the edges. Working from one of the long sides, roll the dough up as tightly as you can into a sausage shape. Cut crosswise into 12 equal pieces.

7 Line a 9 × 13-inch baking pan with parchment paper. Arrange the buns, cut-side up, in the pan, making sure that the tails of the buns are tucked in so they don't unfurl when baked. Allow space around the buns, as they will expand.

8 Cover loosely and leave to rise until the buns are puffed and touching at the sides, 45 minutes to 1 hour. Meanwhile, preheat the oven to 400°F.

9 Bake the buns until golden, about 30 minutes.

10 MEANWHILE, MAKE THE FROSTING: In a bowl, with an electric mixer, beat the cream cheese, butter, orange extract, and orange zest until creamy. Gradually mix in the powdered sugar until blended and smooth.

11 Spread the frosting evenly over the cooled buns. Dust with matcha powder and sprinkle with chopped pistachios.

For the LOVE of CRAB CAKES

It was winter, we were off the road for a spell with the whole family back in Austin. Sister Bobbie lived down the street and I often went over to her place for lunch. She was a great cook who loved making the meals we grew up on.

One year, a brutal ice storm held us up for days. To keep from going stir-crazy, she and I started making music. She was a natural. Her fingers ran over the keys in a special kind of way.

I took Trigger and started picking out a melody. It all came together in less than a half hour.

For lunch that day, she went to the kitchen to cook up the crab cakes that Mama Nelson had made for us as kids. She knew the recipe by heart. The taste of that dish brought back a flood of good memories of when life was a lot simpler than it is today.

Talking about today, here's a brand-new recipe for crab cakes.

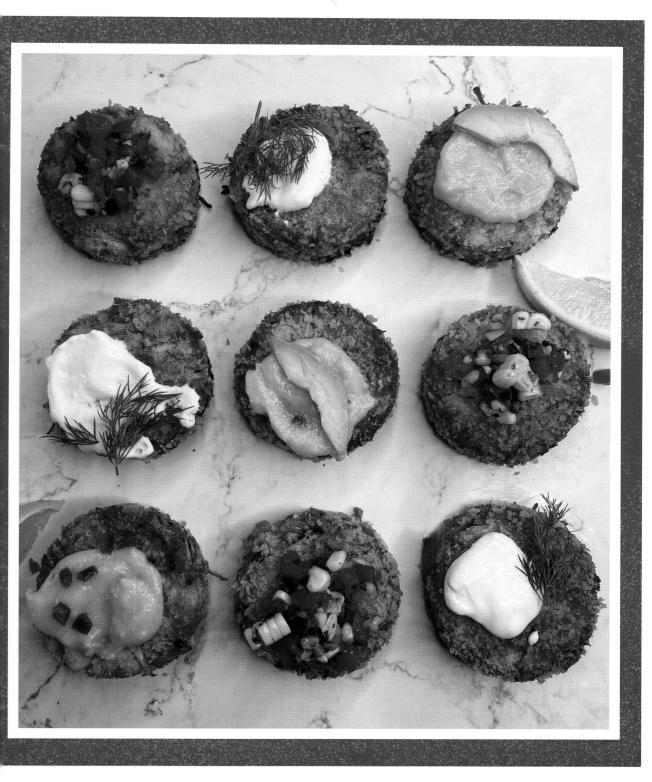

VEGAN CRAB CAKES WITH MANGO JALAPEÑO BUTTER

MAKES **12 CRAB CAKES**
ADD **7.4 MG** PER SERVING IF USING
THE MANGO JALAPEÑO BUTTER

1 (14-ounce) can young green jackfruit, drained

1 (14-ounce) can hearts of palm, drained

1 teaspoon Cannabis Avocado Oil (page 10) or Cannabis Grapeseed Oil (page 11)

2 tablespoons finely diced onion

⅓ cup vegan mayonnaise

1 teaspoon Dijon mustard

3 to 4 tablespoons fresh thyme leaves, minced

1 tablespoon chopped fresh mint

1½ teaspoons chopped fresh parsley

1½ teaspoons garlic powder

1 teaspoon Cajun seasoning

1 teaspoon kosher salt

4 cups panko bread crumbs

4 tablespoons Just Egg (or other egg replacer to equal 1 egg)

1 quart canola or other neutral oil, for frying

Mango Jalapeño Butter (recipe follows), for serving

1 Squeeze excess moisture from the jackfruit and pull it into strands. Chop the hearts of palm into small pieces akin to lump crab.

2 In a medium skillet, heat the cannabis oil over medium heat. Add the onion and cook until slightly translucent.

3 Add the jackfruit and hearts of palm and sauté for an additional 3 to 5 minutes until warmed. Do not allow the ingredients to get mushy.

4 Remove from the heat and transfer to a bowl. Refrigerate until the mixture is thoroughly chilled.

5 Add the mayonnaise, mustard, chopped herbs, garlic powder, Cajun seasoning, and kosher salt. Add 2 cups of the panko and adjust seasoning if needed. Add the egg replacer and mix thoroughly with impeccably clean or gloved hands.

6 Divide the mixture into 6 equal portions and form into patties. Coat the patties in the remaining panko. Set on a plate and refrigerate for 30 minutes to firm up.

7 Meanwhile, heat the oil in a large pot to 350°F. Set a wire rack in a sheet pan and place near the stove.

8 Working in batches of 3, fry the crab cakes until golden brown. Drain on the wire rack.

9 Serve each crab cake with 2 tablespoons mango jalapeño butter.

MANGO JALAPEÑO BUTTER

YIELDS **3½ CUPS**
SERVING SIZE **4½ TABLESPOONS**
10 MG PER SERVING

7½ tablespoons
vegan butter

½ teaspoon Vegan
Cannabis Butter
(page 9)

1 jalapeño, seeded
and chopped

1 shallot, finely
chopped

3 cups diced mango

Kosher salt

1 teaspoon agave
syrup (optional)

1 In a skillet, melt the vegan butter and vegan cannabis butter over medium heat. Add the jalapeño and shallot and cook until softened, about 3 to 5 minutes. Add the mango and cook for an additional 3 to 5 minutes until warm.

2 Season to taste with salt. Add agave for desired sweetness (optional).

3 Transfer to a bowl and use an immersion blender to puree until smooth. Store in the refrigerator.

HAPPY TRAILS

If you're old enough to remember it, "Happy Trails" was the theme song that Roy Rogers and his wife, Dale, sang in two-part harmony, first on their radio show and then on TV. This was back in the forties and fifties when I was trying to figure out how to make a living by making music.

That song got to me. It was simple and sincere. I took it to mean that at some point you have to make a choice. All my choices haven't been good. I've wandered down some sad trails. I've even found myself on dangerous trails. Today, though, I'm pleased to say that, in this golden period, I'm walking a

PPY
ILS

trail that couldn't be better. Fact is, I'm happier than ever.

Much credit for that happiness goes to my wife, Annie, who has shown me how eating healthy food has boosted my energy and enriched the quality of my life, even in my nineties!

I'm proud and pleased that this cookbook shows how healthy food containing cannabis is both creative and delicious.

And I'm hoping that as I wish you happy trails, you'll find even more happiness—and good health—by trying a bunch of these recipes.

See you at the next show.